9.95

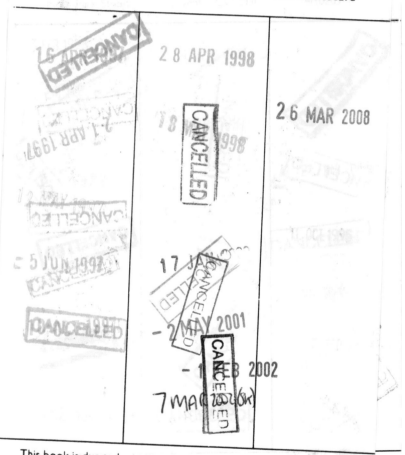

Survey of
FUNCTIONAL
NEUROANATOMY

Second Edition

Survey of FUNCTIONAL NEUROANATOMY

Second Edition

Bill Garoutte, PhD, MD
Professor of Anatomy and Neurology
University of California, San Francisco

JONES MEDICAL PUBLICATIONS — Greenbrae, CA

Distributed by
YEAR BOOK MEDICAL PUBLISHERS
35 East Wacker Drive, Chicago, IL 60601

Copyright © 1987 by Jones Medical Publications

Spanish edition: *Neuroanatomia Funcional.*
Editorial El Manual Moderno, S.A., Mexico, D.F.

Portuguese edition: *Neuroanatomia Funcional.*
Guanabara Koogan, Rio de Janiro, R.J., Brazil.

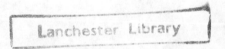
Library of Congress Catalog Number: 87-80375
ISBN: 0-930010-13-2

Printed in USA
0987654321

Jones Medical Publications
355 Los Cerros Drive
Greenbrae, CA 94904

Preface to the First Edition

This book has been developed over a period of years to fill the need of health science professionals for a concise, practical, and up-to-date introduction to the structure of the human nervous system. Biological structure lacks meaning without function, so structure and function have been presented together and related to human patients. This thread of clinical significance appears throughout the book.

Basic scientific aspects of human nervous system structure and function cannot be divorced from clinical aspects. In modern medicine, even the most basic and abstruse of experimental observations relate directly to diseases of human patients.

Clinical examples in each chapter offer opportunities for practice in the sort of human neurobiological analysis that health science professionals use daily. These clinical examples, as well as the text and illustrations, are simplified representatives of events which occur in the real world of human patients. As learning devices the various concepts and processes are presented in isolation, but it must be kept in mind that they **never** occur in isolation in the living body. Every one of these processes goes on within the human nervous system simultaneously and continuously. Lists of study questions appended to each chapter emphasize the important concepts and review the complex vocabulary introduced in the chapter.

Helpfulness and kindness have been my experience throughout the development of this book. First I wish to acknowledge my debt to the hundreds of medical students and physical therapy students who have patiently (at times a bit impatiently) borne the writing and rewriting of the book. To Jack de Groot, from whom I have borrowed unstintingly and who has graciously permitted the borrowing, my thanks for a pleasant and long-lasting association. To the late Ralph Hawkins, strict neuroanatomist, and meticulous neurosurgeon, and valued friend, belated but sincere thanks. Thanks also to Michael Aminoff for thoughtful comments on a late draft of the manuscript, and to Ms Joan Mello for typing the manuscript. Finally, I am grateful for the support of my publisher Richard C. M. Jones, who has deftly guided my efforts through the throes of book production with gentleness, understanding, and insight.

BCG

Preface to the Second Edition

It has been a pleasure to receive the numerous thoughtful comments and suggestions regarding the first edition from colleagues, reviewers, and students. Many of these comments are reflected in the revision, and I hope this will make the book even more valuable and useful to students of the structure and function of the human nervous system.

San Francisco
March, 1987
BCG

Contents

1 General Overview of the Human CNS

The human central nervous system (CNS) consists of the brain and spinal cord. The former a complex collection of more that a trillion neurons (gray matter) and of multitudinous nerve fibers (white matter) within the bony cranial cavity, and the latter within the spinal column. These numerous neurons interact through an even larger number (10^{15} or more) of interconnections (synapses). The CNS forms the morphologic and functional unit that mediates awareness, defines personality and individuality, perceives the world around us, and controls our responses to it.

In vertebrates less complex than humans, the CNS may have a tubular form. With the cephalization (increasing importance of the head) of *Homo sapiens,* the rostral end of the neural tube has enlarged and become much more complex, forming cerebrum, cerebellum, and other cephalic neural structures. The spinal cord of humans has retained a roughly cylindrical configuration.

Collections of neuronal cell bodies within the CNS are called nuclei, each usually subsuming restricted functions. Processes or extensions of neuronal bodies, called axons, collect together into bundles of nerve fibers called tracts. Most of neurobiology is encompassed in the identification of nuclei and tracts and their functions.

The major subdivisions of the human CNS are as follows and can be identified in Figures 1-7.

SPINAL CORD   An elongated cylindrical structure lying within the spinal canal and extending 35-50 cm from the foramen magnum of the skull to the level of the second lumbar vertebra (L2).

MEDULLA   An expanded rostral extension of the spinal cord through the foramen magnum, lying within the posterior fossa of the cranial cavity. Length about 4 cm.

PONS and CEREBELLUM occupy the remainder of the posterior fossa. Many of the structures of the medulla continue rostrally through the pons.

MIDBRAIN (mesencephalon) is a rostral continuation of the pons. It is the uppermost part of the brain stem, and lies in the incisura (notch) of the tentorium which separates the posterior fossa (infratentorial compartment) from the supratentorial compartment of the cranial cavity.

DIENCEPHALON   In the adult, this subdivision of the CNS consists of a complex collection of nuclei lying symmetrically on either side of the midline third ventricle in the depths of the cerebrum. It can be usefully divided into four major components (thalamus, hypothalamus, epithalamus, subthalamus), of which the thalamus is the largest (see Figure 22).

CEREBRUM (telencephalon)   Two hemispheres, surrounding the diencephalon and consisting of basal ganglia in the depths of the cerebrum, and the cerebral cortex, which is the layer of neurons on the surface. Between them, large masses of axons (nerve fibers = white matter) provide elaborate inter-connections to, from, and between cortical neurons.

These subdivisions of the CNS fall naturally into an hierarchy, with the spinal cord lowest and the cerebral cortex, seat of consciousness, usually accorded the highest level.

Through its spinal nerves, the spinal cord bears sensory information from the periphery, and sends motor impulses toward the same peripheral regions. Many reflex mechanisms act directly through the spinal cord, connecting sensory inputs with motor outputs without involving higher levels.

Brain stem usually refers to medulla, pons, and midbrain as a unit. The brain stem continues the structure of the spinal cord rostrally, and mediates for the face the kinds of functions carried by the spinal cord for the rest of the body. Further, within the brain stem, lie most of the auditory and vestibular (hearing and equilibratory) and oculomotor (eye movement) systems. These complex functions make possible the minute resolution and accuracy of our two major senses, vision and hearing.

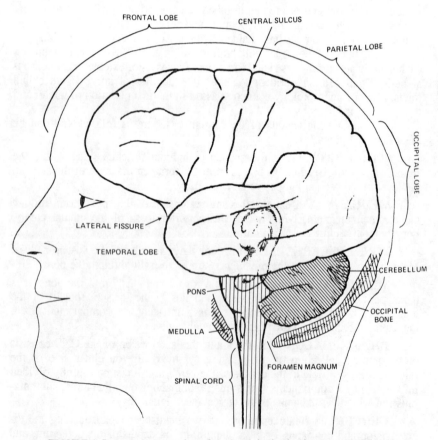

FIGURE 1. Lateral phantom view of the head, indicating important landmarks

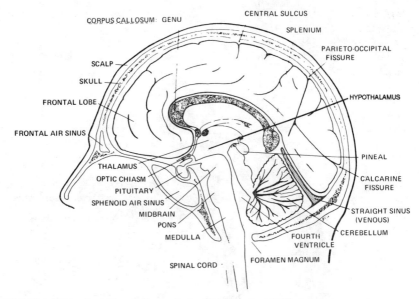

FIGURE 2. Midsagittal view of the head, showing important CNS structures

The cerebellum, in large part a phylogenetically new organ, coordinates volitional motor functions. From the pons, as well as from medulla and spinal cord, sensory and other information come to the cerebellum via large and important tracts, to take part in these coordinating functions.

Paired collections of nuclei consisting of billions of neurons make up the four divisions of the diencephalon. Nuclei of the thalamus relay sensory, motor, and other impulses to the cerebral cortex, and interact with the cortex. The hypothalamus controls endocrine functions and many of the basic (vegetative) life processes, such as assimilation of food and water, reproductive functions, and control of electrolytes and temperature. Ventral to the caudal end of the thalamus lies a collection of nuclei, the subthalamus, mostly concerned with motor functions. Epithalamus refers, in the human, to a small group of dorsal nuclei with unknown functions, the habenula, and part of the pineal gland. Because of their connections, they are usually lumped with the limbic system (see Chapter 17).

Basal ganglia, including caudate nucleus, lentiform nucleus (putamen and globus pallidus), and several smaller nuclei, also act as ancillary motor systems, receiving information from the cortex and other sources, and feeding back to the motor areas of the cortex.

On the convoluted surface of the cerebrum, a layer of neurons 3-5 mm thick constitutes the cerebral cortex. At about 50,000 neurons/square mm of surface area, the cortex includes approximately fifteen billion neurons, and mediates all the functions of humans ordinarily described as sapient. These can be subsumed under the general rubric of symbolic functions. Included are language in all its manifestations, memory, logical and illogical thought, geometric, geographic, and self perception, and volitional control of many of the body's functions.

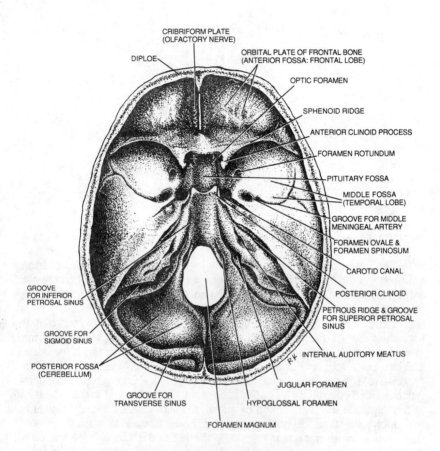

CRIBRIFORM PLATE
(OLFACTORY NERVE)

DIPLOE

ORBITAL PLATE OF FRONTAL BONE
(ANTERIOR FOSSA: FRONTAL LOBE)

OPTIC FORAMEN

SPHENOID RIDGE

ANTERIOR CLINOID PROCESS

FORAMEN ROTUNDUM

PITUITARY FOSSA

MIDDLE FOSSA
(TEMPORAL LOBE)

GROOVE FOR MIDDLE
MENINGEAL ARTERY

FORAMEN OVALE &
FORAMEN SPINOSUM

CAROTID CANAL

POSTERIOR CLINOID

PETROUS RIDGE & GROOVE
FOR SUPERIOR PETROSAL
SINUS

INTERNAL AUDITORY MEATUS

JUGULAR FORAMEN

HYPOGLOSSAL FORAMEN

FORAMEN MAGNUM

GROOVE FOR
TRANSVERSE SINUS

POSTERIOR FOSSA
(CEREBELLUM)

GROOVE FOR
SIGMOID SINUS

GROOVE
FOR INFERIOR
PETROSAL SINUS

FIGURE 3. Floor of the cranial cavity
(Drawing by Dr. Rebecca Kasten.)

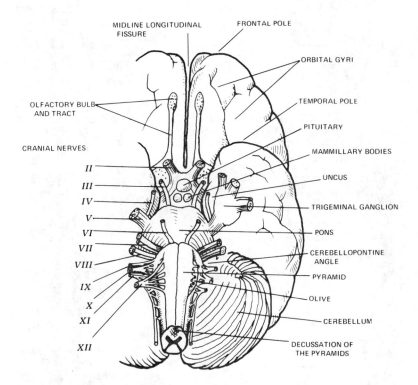

FIGURE 4. Base of the brain showing the twelve cranial nerves. (Modified from drawing by Ms Lena Lyons, reproduced with permission of the artist and Dr. Jack De Groot.) See also Figures 96 and 97 for other views of the brain stem.

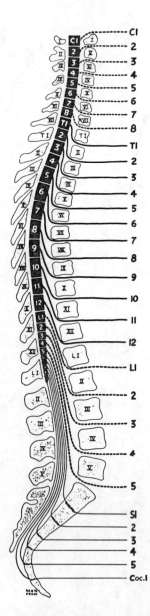

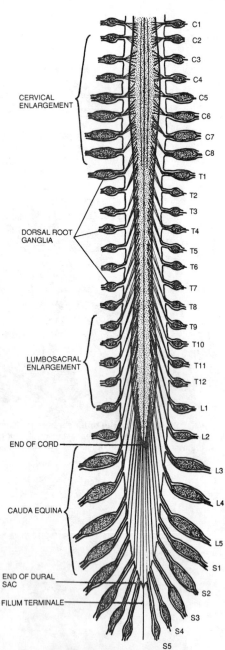

FIGURE 5. Sagittal section of spinal cord and vertebral column, showing relationship of nerve roots. (Reproduced with permission, from Haymaker & Woodhall: *Peripheral Nerve Injuries*, Saunders, 1956.)

FIGURE 6. Dorsal view of spinal cord and dural sac, with plan of roots and dorsal root ganglia. Note the large size of dorsal root ganglia and the cord at cervical and lumbosacral levels, associated with the high density innervations of hands and feet.

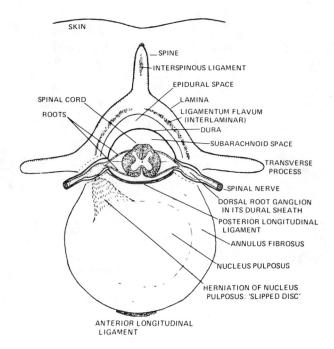

FIGURE 7. Cross-section of spine, showing relationship of spinal cord and dura.

STUDY QUESTIONS

1. Name and identify, both in illustrations and on gross brain specimens, the major subdivisions of the human CNS.

2. What are the anterior, middle, and posterior cranial fossae? Identify them in illustrations and on a dried human skull.

3. What lie in these fossae during life?

4. What is the cerebral cortex? Identify it in illustrations and gross specimens.

5. What is meant by white matter in the CNS?

6. What is meant by gray matter?

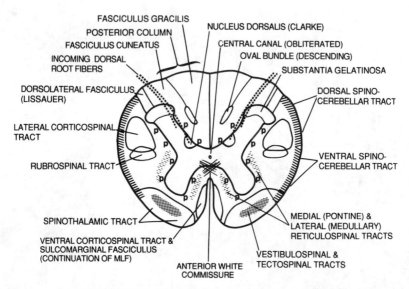

FIGURE 8. Major structures of the human spinal cord, diagrammatic.
P = Propriospinal bundles = Fasciculus proprius

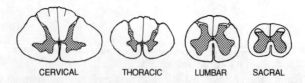

CERVICAL   THORACIC   LUMBAR   SACRAL

FIGURE 9. Cross-sections of the spinal cord at representative levels. Note the oval shape and large anterior horns of the cervical cord, the thin gray columns and the lateral horn of the thoracic cord, and the increasing volume of white matter (nerve fibers—axons) as one proceeds rostrally. (Compare also Figures 8 and 72.)

2 Neuroembryology

In its earliest development, the human zygote differs little from frogs or chicks, either in form or in sequence of changes. Evolutionary modifications soon become apparent, however, and some stages prominent in lower forms are missing in the human. Just after the human zygote and its associated cells implant in the wall of the uterus, two cavities appear, the endodermal vesicle and the ectodermal vesicle. The flattened embryonal plate interposed between the two vesicles consists of the classical three layers: ectoderm, endoderm, and mesoderm. Here develops the embryo (see Figure 10).

About the middle of the first month of gestation, the ectodermal layer of the embryonal plate begins to fold up into two parallel longitudinal ridges, the neural folds (Figure 11). The neural folds grow both longitudinally and vertically, eventually folding over and fusing to form the neural tube (Figures 12A and B). Fusion occurs first at the level that will be midcervical in the adult, and proceeds both rostrally and caudally. Final closure of the anterior neuropore, at the level of the lamina terminalis, and of the posterior neuropore, at a lumbosacral spinal cord level, occurs about the end of the first month (see Table 2).

Failures of the neural tube to close completely cause common congenital malformations: Myelocele (myel = spinal cord; cele = cavity), the most serious of these malformations, results from lack of fusion of the neural folds, so that dura, vertebral arch, and skin are all missing and the spinal cord remains exposed. Because of unavoidable infection, this malformation is not usually compatible with life. In meningoceles, the skin and vertebral arch are incomplete. The dura is exposed dorsally, covering and protecting the cord. Though the cord may be defective in such babies, survival is possible if the skin can be closed by plastic surgery. In spina bifida, only the bony vertebral arch fails to fuse, but skin and dura are intact. This usually causes no symptoms.

All the complex structures of the adult brain and spinal cord develop from the primordial neural tube. In the angle between the developing neural tube and the overlying ectoderm, a line of cells differentiates from the neural tube, this is the neural crest (Figure 12B). From these cells arise a number of important peripheral neurectodermal derivatives, listed in Table 3.

Forebrain, midbrain, and hindbrain vesicles, characteristic of lower forms, never appear as such in human CNS development. During the rapid and complex multiplication of cells forming the primordia of adult brain structures, this three-vesicle stage does not occur. By the fourth week, most adult structures can be identified, though often only as groups of primitive neuroblast cells (Figure 13).

In early development, the human brain forms three bends or flexures: cephalic, pontine, and cervical. They occur respectively at the midbrain level, at

TABLE 1. Embryonic subdivisions of the human CNS

Embryonic divisions		Adult derivatives	Ventricular cavities
Forebrain (Prosencephalon) {	Telencephalon {	Cerebral cortex Basal ganglia	Lateral ventricles
	Diencephalon {	Thalamus Hypothalamus Subthalamus Epithalamus	Third ventricle
Midbrain (Mesencephalon)	----	{ Tectum Cerebral peduncles	Aqueduct
Hindbrain (Rhombencephalon) {	Metencephalon {	Cerebellum Pons	Fourth ventricle
	Myelencephalon	Medulla	
Spinal cord	---	Spinal cord	No cavity

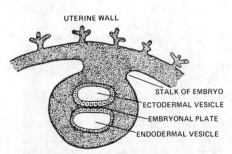

FIGURE 10. The embryonal plate lies between the primitive vesicles at the time of implantation.

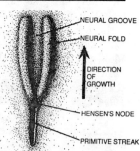

FIGURE 11. View of the neuronal folds on the ectodermal aspect of the embryonal plate. (Drawing by Dr. Rebecca Kasten.)

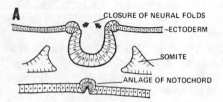

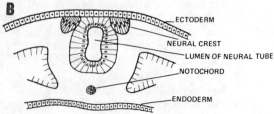

FIGURE 12. Closure of neural folds to form neural tube. (A) Just before closure. (B) Just after. Somites are the framework of bony structures. Neural crest cells migrate peripherally. The notochord is essential to normal development, and eventually lies in the center of the adult vertebral body.

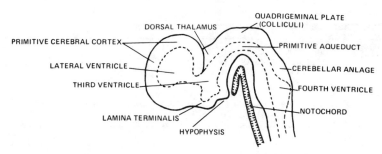

FIGURE 13. Week 4. Lateral view of the CNS. Primitive ventricular cavities shown thus - - -

TABLE 2. Brief timetable of human prenatal brain development.

What happens?		Length	Age
First cell division			30-60 hrs
100-cell blastocyst			5 days
Implantation			
Notochord anlage; first blood islands		0.45 mm	7 days
	Somites		
Neural tube closure starts	5	2 mm	22 days
Cephalic and cervical flexures; Gill arches; Rathke's pouch	15	2.6	25 days
Anterior neuropore closes; optic and otic vesicles	25	3.5 mm	27 days
Posterior neuropore closes	30		30 days
Upper limb bud; olfactory, optic cups		5 mm	35 days
Cerebral vesicle; pontine flexure; face fusing		9 mm	41 days
Hypophysis fusing		11 mm	45 days
Choroid plexus; fibers into optic chiasm		17 mm	47 days
Cerebellar rudiment; insula appearing		27 mm	55 days
First reflex to skin touch (face)			56 days
Anterior and hippocampal commissures		30 mm	60 days
First 'spontaneous' movement; palate fusing		35 mm	70 days
Calcarine fissure; corpus callosum		50 mm	2.5 mos
	Weight of fetus		
Cervical flexure flattened	20 gm	55 mm	3 mos
Foramen of Magendie; primordium of cortex	120 gm	100 mm	4 mos
First myelin; motor cranial nerves	300 gm	150 mm	5 mos
Myelination in MLF	600 gm	350 mm	6 mos
Optic and pyramidal myelination begin	3000 gm	350 mm	10 mos

Note: These figures are averages; there is much individual variation.

TABLE 3. Adult cells which develop from the neural crest

1. Dorsal root ganglia
2. Sympathetic (paravertebral) ganglia
3. Other ganglia of the autonomic nervous system
4. Medulla of the adrenal gland
5. Chromaffin cells in the gut and elsewhere
6. Melanophores; pigment-containing cells in skin, hair, eye and elsewhere
7. Schwann cells of peripheral nerve

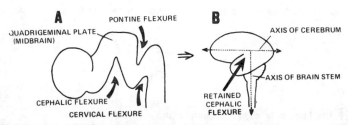

FIGURE 14. Embryonic flexures of the human brain. (A) At 6 weeks' gestation. (B) Adult. Pontine flexure appears at 6 weeks and is lost at 4 months. Cervical flexure appears at 3 weeks and is lost at 4 months. Cephalic flexure appears at 3 weeks at the level of the midbrain, and is retained to adulthood.

the pons, and between medulla and cord. Only the cephalic flexure remains in the adult, so that the long axis of the adult cerebrum is horizontal, while the brain stem is at right angles, nearly vertical (Figure 14).

Figure 15A, B, C illustrates the tremendous changes in form and size of the cerebral hemisphere and its cavity, the lateral ventricle. Cortical convolutions (sulci and gyri) appear late in gestation, and are not sketched in Figure 15.

Table 2 briefly summarizes the sequence of CNS development. The changes tabulated result from proliferation, migration, and the normal processes of cell death that characterize specific groups of neurons. Such timetables provide clues to the effects of prenatal insults to the embryo, because structures developing rapidly at a given instant are particularly susceptible to damage, whatever the cause of the damage (infection, trauma, intoxications, anoxia, etc.) As deduced from Table 2, the first two to three months of intrauterine life (the first trimester) are particularly important in this respect.

Contemporaneous with the gross changes listed in Table 2, microscopic and submicroscopic development of synaptic connections between neurons (synaptogenesis) occurs. Disruption of the processes of synaptogenesis probably accounts for congenital defects, such as mental subnormality, where no gross defect can be identified.

CLINICAL EXAMPLE 1

A woman who had been a known alcoholic for years delivered a baby with meningocele (nonclosure of the neural tube) and severe mental defect, together with cardiac malformations. Discuss

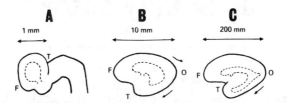

FIGURE 15. Development of cerebral hemispheres and lateral ventricles. (A) 1 month (compare Figure 14). (B) 3 months. (C) Adult (compare Figures 1 and 2). F = frontal lobe. O = occipital lobe. T = temporal lobe.

Discussion

Ethyl alcohol is much more toxic to the fetus (and to the very young child) than to adults. This patient probably binged on alcohol during the first trimester of gestation. The resultant toxic levels of blood alcohol crossed the placenta and deranged the cellular development of neural and cardiac structures.

STUDY QUESTIONS

1. Tumors containing skin and hair (dermoids) occasionally occur in the CNS of children. Account for this on embryologic grounds.
2. Toxins, infections, etc., may cause maldevelopment of the CNS. The specific maldevelopment depends on which structures are actively developing at the time of the insult. Using Table 2, what congenital malformations might you expect if an infection occurred at 1 month? At 2 months?
3. What is a meningocele?
4. What is spina bifida?
5. What is the neural crest?

3 Blood Supply of the CNS

Stroke, meaning damage to the CNS from blockage or other disruption of parts of its blood supply, constitutes the third largest cause of death in the United States (see Table 4).

TABLE 4. Leading causes of death in the USA (1978 census data)

1.	Heart disease	729,510
2.	Cancer	396,992
3.	Strokes	175,629
4.	Accidents	105,561

Degeneration of nervous tissue (infarction) results from interruption of blood supply as brief as 10 minutes. Neurons themselves can often survive up to 30 minutes without blood, but the lack of glucose and oxygen causes permanent capillary occlusion from swelling of the endothelial lining of cerebral capillaries after only a few minutes without blood.

As an indication of the brain's high metabolic requirements, it makes up only 2 percent of the adult's body weight, but needs 10-20 percent of cardiac output. It uses 20 percent of the body's oxygen consumption and up to 66 percent of the liver's glucose production.

ARTERIAL CIRCLE OF WILLIS

An anastomotic group of arteries at the base of the brain, the circle of Willis, is the key to understanding the blood supply to the brain. Two internal carotid arteries and two vertebral arteries supply blood to the arterial circle, which in turn distributes it to all intracranial nervous structures (Figures 16, 17, and 20).

THE SYSTEM OF THE INTERNAL CAROTID ARTERY

Internal and external carotid arteries originate from the common carotid artery in the neck. The external carotid supplies face, scalp, and other extracranial structures. It only rarely supplies intracranial nervous structures, and then by way of anomalous or abnormal connections. The internal carotid artery enters the cranial cavity through the carotid canal in the floor of the middle cranial fossa. The artery passes forward through the cavernous sinus just lateral to the pituitary fossa (sella turcica), then bends upward into the cranial cavity medial to the anterior clinoid process (see Figures 3, 17, and 20).

It terminates shortly after entering the cranial cavity, branching into the middle cerebral artery and the anterior cerebral artery (Figures 16 and 18B). The former sends perforating arteries into the base of the cerebrum to supply internal structures, then passes laterally to supply the cortex of the lateral convexity of the cerebrum (Figures 18, 20, and 21). Deep perforating arteries

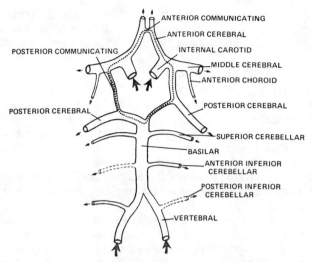

FIGURE 16. Arterial circle of Willis, indicated by dotted lines. Inferior cerebellar arteries are inconstant (dotted lines). On the left side, the posterior cerebral artery arises from the basilar. In about one-third of hemispheres, it arises from the internal carotid, as shown on the right side of the sketch. Arrows indicate direction of blood flow.

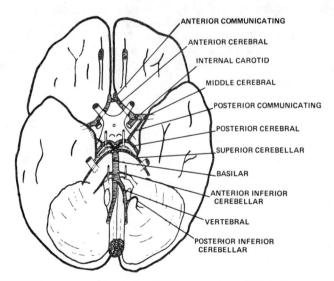

FIGURE 17. The arteries of the circle of Willis on the base of the brain.

also arise from the anterior cerebral artery. It then supplies the frontal lobe and loops around the front (genu) of the corpus callosum to provide blood for superior cortical areas as far back as the parietal lobe (Figures 18A and 21A,B).

VERTEBROBASILAR SYSTEM

Each vertebral artery in the neck ascends through the transverse foramina of the upper six cervical vertebrae, then loops backward and upward around the atlas (first cervical vertebra) to pierce the dura and enter the cranial cavity through the foramen magnum (Figure 19A). Shortly after entering the cranial cavity, the vertebral artery gives off the posterior inferior cerebellar artery (PICA) which supplies the inferior part of the cerebellum, the lateral third of the medulla and the choroid plexus of the fourth ventricle. The vertebral arteries of the two sides then fuse anterior to the medulla to form the basilar artery (Figures 16, 17, and 19B).

Additional blood supply to the cerebellum arises from the basilar artery, anterior inferior cerebellar arteries, and superior cerebellar arteries. Numerous small pontine perforating arteries arise from the basilar to supply the pons.

At the rostral border of the pons, the basilar artery terminates by branching into the two posterior cerebral arteries, which also send deep perforating branches into the cerebrum (Figure 20). They then pass backward around the cerebral peduncles, which they supply. Small branches supply deep midbrain structures, including the reticular activating system (RAS), whose function is the maintenance of consciousness. The posterior cerebrals continue backward to supply the occipital lobe, giving off en route branches which supply the choroid plexuses of the third and lateral ventricles.

As commented earlier, occlusion of the cerebral artery results in infarction of a volume of nervous tissue. Because any artery, large or small, can be occluded, many types of neurological disturbances can result from such infarction, depending on its specific size and location.

ARTERIAL ANASTOMOSES

In addition to the circle of Willis, many small anastomotic channels occur in the brain. Anastomotic arteries allow blood flow across the boundaries between the principal areas supplied by the large branches of the circle of Willis, as well as between superficial and deep areas of supply. These anastomoses often restrict the area of infarction to a small portion of the region normally supplied by the occluded vessel (see Figure 21C).

PERFORATING OR BASAL ARTERIES

All the brain's blood vessels develop embryologically in the pia on the surface, and the large vessels remain there in the adult. Arteriolar branches with muscular walls leave the large surface vessels to perforate the brain at right angles and supply deep structures. Blood pressure in the large surface vessels is high, close to cardiac output pressure. The muscular walls of the perforating arterioles control the blood flow to local areas of the brain, a process called 'autoregulation.' Larger perforating branches, taking off the basilar artery or the circle of Willis supply pons, deep structures of the brainstem, basal ganglia, thalamus, hypothalamus, internal capsule, ands other internal structures (see Figures 20 and 22).

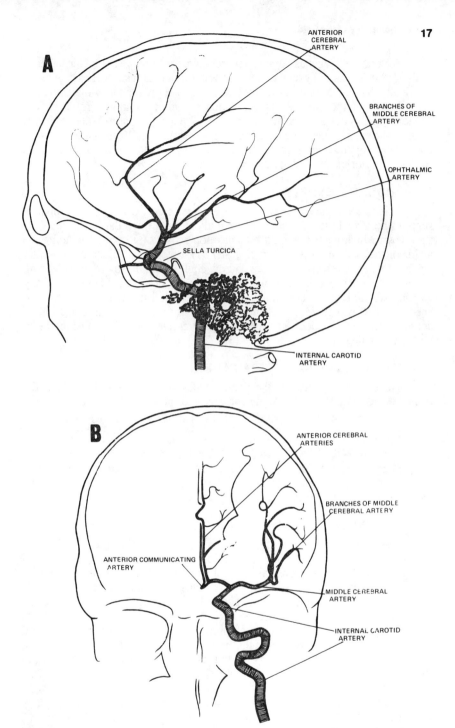

FIGURE 18. Carotid arteriography. (A) Lateral view, arterial phase. (B) Anteroposterior view, arterial phase. Both anterior cerebral arteries were filled in this instance via the anterior communicating artery.

Perforating branches of the anterior cerebral artery supply the anterior limb of the internal capsule as well as anterior thalamus and basal ganglia. Lenticulostriate arteries from the middle cerebral supply anterior thalamus and central parts of the internal capsule, often including motor fibers. Their occlusion causes contralateral hemiplegia. They enter the base of the cerebrum through the anterior perforated substance just behind the olfactory tract. Posterior perforating (thalamic) branches plunge into the interpeduncular fossa, to supply posterior thalamus and adjacent structures.

MIDDLE MENINGEAL ARTERY

This is a periosteal branch of the external carotid artery and ordinarily supplies no CNS tissue. It enters the cranial cavity through the foramen spinosum, from which point it and its branches form a set of grooves ascending the inside of the skull vault (see Figures 3 and 31). It becomes clinically important when ruptured by fracture of the lateral skull vault, followed by bleeding between dura and overlying skull. This extradural or epidural hematoma may develop slowly over several hours or days, even after apparent recovery from head injury. If recognized, the hematoma is easily removed by trephination. If not recognized, the patient may die from progressive compression of the brain by the expanding clot.

VENOUS DRAINAGE OF THE BRAIN

Three major systems of the dural venous sinuses drain blood from the cranial contents into the internal jugular veins, for return to the heart:

1. The system of the superior sagittal sinus (SSS) — Figures 23 and 24.
2. The galenic system — Figure 23.
3. The system of the cavernous sinus — Figure 23.

Dural venous sinuses are endothelium-lined venous channels surrounded by dura. Neither sinuses nor other cerebral veins possess valves, so that the blood flows in either direction, depending on momentary pressures.

GALENIC SYSTEM OF VEINS

The great cerebral vein of Galen is usually only 1 cm in length, lies just behind and under the splenium of the corpus callosum in the midline, and drains the interior of the cerebral hemispheres. It is formed by the junction of the two internal cerebral veins, each of which drains one hemisphere via terminal (thalamostriate), septal, and choroidal veins (Figure 23). Right and left basal veins, draining the base of the cerebrum anteriorly, also empty into the great cerebral vein. The great vein empties into the straight sinus in the dural junction between falx cerebri and the two leaves of the tentorium (Figure 31). Blood flows backward in the straight sinus and in the superior sagittal sinus, to the confluence. The SSS is ordinarily the larger vessel, draining via the confluence into the right transverse sinus (Figure 24) thence into the right internal jugular vein. Blood from the straight sinus drains to the left. In many individuals the two streams mix at the confluence.

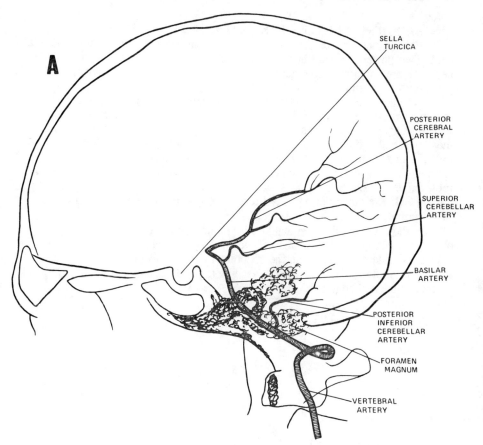

FIGURE 19A. Right vertebral arteriography. Lateral view — anterior inferior cerebellar not filled.

EMISSARY VEINS

In addition to the major venous drainage via the internal jugular veins (Figures 23 and 24), a variable number of smaller veins pierce the skull to connect dural venous sinuses with extracranial veins. The ophthalmic vein (Figure 23) exemplifies this, connecting the cavernous sinus with facial veins. Similar veins pass through most of the cranial foramina, accompanying cranial nerves and arteries, and there are usually a few which pierce the skull directly: parietal emissary veins; posterior condylar veins.

As they are without valves, emissary veins provide emergency drainage when the internal jugular veins are occluded. They also assume clinical importance as pathways for entrance of extracranial infections, from scalp, face, ear, or neck. Such infections may cause infected thrombosis in venous sinuses. Infected sinus thrombosis was always fatal before discovery and use of antibiotics.

BLOOD SUPPLY OF THE SPINAL CORD

From a network of pial arteries, perforating vessels supply the spinal cord. Two posterior spinal arteries and one anterior spinal artery of the pial network are relatively constant, supplying respectively the dorsolateral quadrants of the cord, and its ventral half (see Figure 25).

Arteries to supply the cord enter the spinal canal through intervertebral foramina in company with spinal nerves. They are called radicular arteries if they supply only nerve roots. If they supply blood both to roots and to cord, they are called radiculospinal arteries. Each radiculospinal artery supplies blood to half a dozen spinal cord segments, with the exception of the large artery of Adamkiewicz, which usually enters with the left second lumbar (L2) ventral root, range T10-L4, and supplies most of the caudal third of the cord (Figures 25 and 26). The upper cervical cord receives blood from the vertebral arteries via recurrent branches.

Radicular and radiculospinal arteries branch off the vertebral in the neck, off intercostals in the thorax, and off the aorta at the abdominal level (Figure 26). Arteriosclerotic changes in the abdominal aorta can occlude these vessels and result in infarction of the cord — leading to paralysis and loss of sensation of lower trunk and both legs.

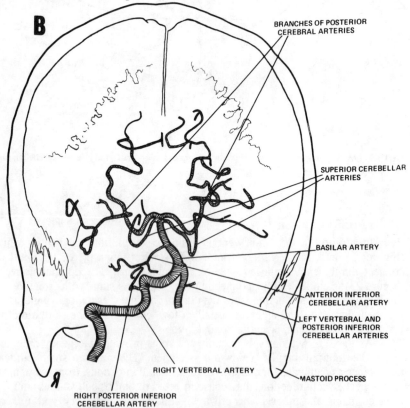

FIGURE 19B. Right vertebral arteriogaphy. Anterioposterior view —note reflux with partial filling of left vertebral and posterior inferior cerebellar arteries.

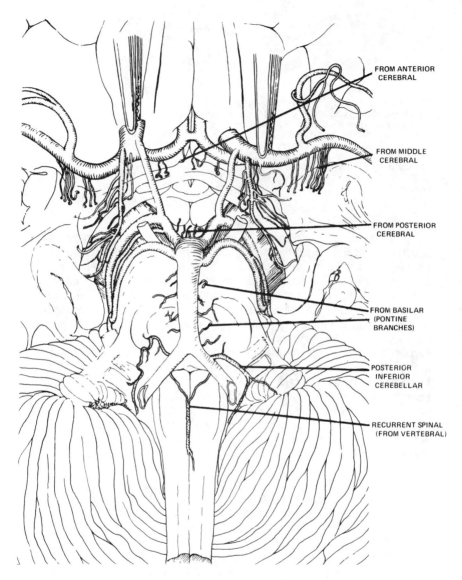

FROM ANTERIOR
CEREBRAL

FROM MIDDLE
CEREBRAL

FROM POSTERIOR
CEREBRAL

FROM BASILAR
(PONTINE
BRANCHES)

POSTERIOR
INFERIOR
CEREBELLAR

RECURRENT SPINAL
(FROM VERTEBRAL)

FIGURE 20. Perforating (central) branches of arteries of the circle of Willis. (Modified from Alexander, L. *in* 'Diseases of the Basal Ganglia' *ARNMD.* 21:71-132, 1942.)

Venous drainage of the spinal cord generally parallels its arterial supply. Large venous channels outside the dura in the spinal canal connect through the foramen magnum with intracranial vessels in the posterior fossa. These connections may extend the length of the spine and may act as a route for spread of infection or carcinoma from pelvic or abdominal organs to the brain.

22 Blood supply of the CNS

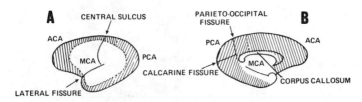

FIGURE 21. Blood supply of cerebral cortex.
(a) Lateral view. ACA, MCA, and PCA =
anterior, middle, and posterior cerebral
arteries. (B) Medial view. (C) Effect of
occlusion of middle cerebral artery. Note
that the infarcted region is smaller than the
MCA's area of supply because of anastomotic blood supply from adjacent
arteries.

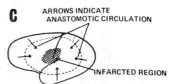

BLOOD-BRAIN BARRIER

When injected intravascularly, large-molecule dyes stain almost all body structures except the brain and nerves. The barrier that prevents the diffusion of proteins, dyes and other substances from blood into the brain parenchyma consists primarily of tight junctions between endothelial cells lining CNS capillaries. In the choroid plexus the situation is different: choroidal capillaries do not possess tight junctions, instead the tight junctions are between the cells of the choroidal epithelium facing the ventricular cavity. Tight junctions between cells of the arachnoid provide the external part of the blood-brain barrier. There is no such barrier in the ventricular walls or pia. Substances in any of the CSF spaces can diffuse freely into the substance of the CNS. A blood-nerve barrier exists in peripheral nerve, made up of tight junctions between the cells of the perineureum surrounding the nerve, and between the endothelial cells of the capillaries supplying the nerve.

Most large molecules and many small molecules which traverse the barrier from blood to brain do so through processes which require metabolic energy, rather than by passive diffusion.

STUDY QUESTIONS

1. Sudden occlusion of one internal carotid or vertebral artery usually causes symptoms, while gradual occlusion, as by developing arteriosclerosis, often does not. Review the circle of Willis, to identify the vessels whose diameters would be likely to increase following such a vascular occlusion. Increases in arterial diameter of course can occur only gradually, which accounts for the importance of time required for the occlusion.

2. Occlusion of any artery or vein may occur, causing infarction of the deprived tissue, and leading to signs and symptoms associated with loss of function of the damaged tissue. Because the student has probably not yet learned specific functions of CNS structures, it is recommended that in subsequent chapters as each structure is discussed, the effects of infarction be reviewed.

3. Identify the CNS regions which would infarct following occlusion of each of the large arteries and veins discussed in this chapter.

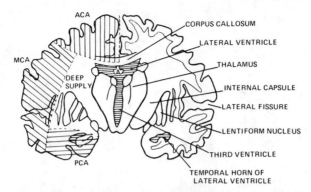

FIGURE 22. Blood supply of cerebrum. Deep structures are supplied by perforating branches from the circle of Willis (see Figure 20). ACA, MCA, and PCA = anterior, middle, and posterior cerebral arteries.

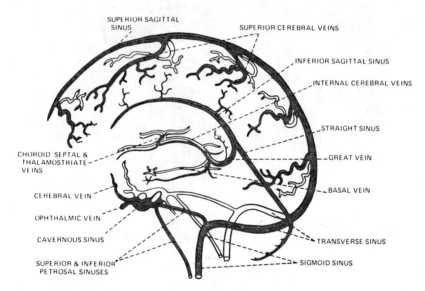

FIGURE 23. Venous drainage of the brain with internal venous channels and the dural venous sinuses. Right sided vessels indicated by unfilled outlines. (Reproduced, courtesy of Eastman Kodak Company.)

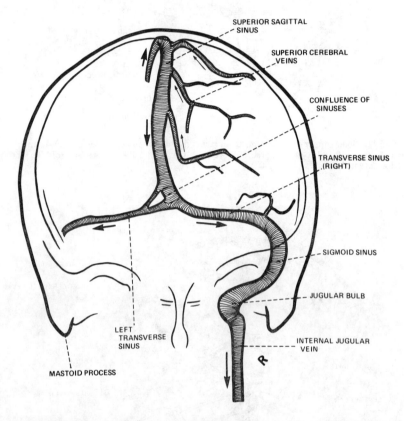

FIGURE 24. Venogram — venous phase of a right carotid arteriogram. Most of the blood from the superior sagittal sinus exits via right transverse sinus and jugular vein.

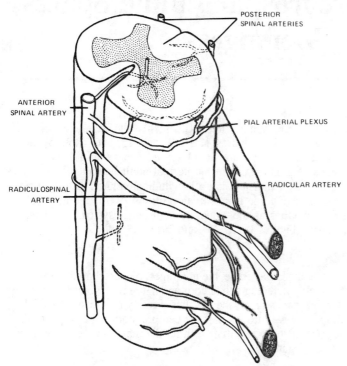

POSTERIOR
SPINAL ARTERIES

ANTERIOR
SPINAL ARTERY

PIAL ARTERIAL PLEXUS

RADICULAR ARTERY

RADICULOSPINAL
ARTERY

FIGURE 25. Arterial blood supply to the spinal cord. (Modified and reproduced, with permission, from Aminoff: *Spinal Angiomas*, Blackwell Scientific Publications, Oxford, 1976.)

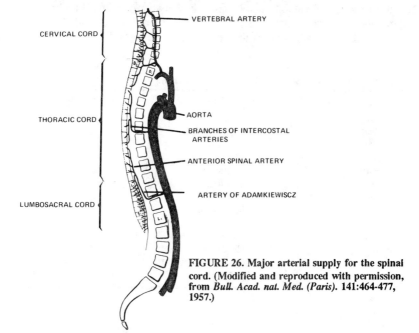

CERVICAL CORD

VERTEBRAL ARTERY

THORACIC CORD

AORTA

BRANCHES OF INTERCOSTAL
ARTERIES

ANTERIOR SPINAL ARTERY

ARTERY OF ADAMKIEWISCZ

LUMBOSACRAL CORD

FIGURE 26. Major arterial supply for the spinal cord. (Modified and reproduced with permission, from *Bull. Acad. nat. Med. (Paris).* 141:464-477, 1957.)

4 Cerebrospinal Fluid Spaces and Meninges

Clear, colorless cerebrospinal fluid (CSF) fills the ventricles of the hollow embryonic neural tube (Figures 12B, 13, and 15, and Table 5), and surrounds the CNS, filling the subarachnoid space. The ventricles are lined with ependyma, cells of glial origin. In the normal adult human spinal cord, there is no lumen, its only remnant being a longitudinal column of ependymal cells in the center of the cord. Intracranial portions of the human CNS, however, retain their cavities as the elaborate ventricular system, lined with ciliated adult ependyma (Figures 15, 27, 28, and 29).

MENINGES

Three layers of connective tissue, the meninges, pia, arachnoid, and dura, surround the entire CNS, including spinal cord and nerve roots, brain stem, and cerebrum. The thin innermost layer, the pia, lies directly on the surface of the nervous tissue, dipping down into sulci of the cerebral cortex, but not into the sulci between the folia of the cerebellum. Within the pial layer lie the arteries and veins of the brain (Figure 30).

CSF SPACES

Next outside and completely investing the pia is the arachnoid, so-called because of a resemblance to a spider's web. Between arachnoid and pia is the subarachnoid space, surrounding brain and spinal cord and filled with cerebrospinal fluid, which also fills the ventricles (Figures 27-30).

TABLE 5. Major constituents of normal CSF and serum

	CSF	Serum
Water	95%	—
Specific gravity	1.007	—
Osmolarity	295 mOsm/liter	295
Sodium	138 mEq/liter	138
Potassium	2.8 mEq/liter	4.1
Calcium	2.4 mEq/liter	5.2
Chloride	124 mEq/liter	101
CO_2 tension	48 mm HG	38(arterial)
pH	7.31	7.41
Glucose	> 45 mg/dl	90
Protein	15 - 50 mg/dl	6.5 - 8.4 gm/dl
Cells	< 5 mm² (lymphocytes)	—
Resting pressure	70-180 mm H_2O	—

CSF DYNAMICS

Choroid plexuses of lateral, third, and fourth ventricles secrete about 75 percent of the CSF (Figure 28). The remainder appears to arise from capillaries in ventricular walls. Choroid plexuses receive their blood supply through three pairs of arteries. A branch of the posterior inferior cerebellar artery (Figure 16) supplies the plexus of the fourth ventricle. A branch of the posterior cerebral artery goes to the third ventricle, and also supplies blood to the upper part of the choroid plexus of the lateral ventricle. Most of the choroid plexus of the lateral ventricle is supplied from below by the anterior choroidal artery (Figure 16), which enters the plexus in the temporal horn of the lateral ventricle. Total CSF flow in the adult averages about 500 ml/day. The fluid flows caudally through the system of ventricles finally exiting from the fourth ventricle via three apertures, the lateral and midline apertures of Luschka and Magendie, to enter the cisterna magna, an area of widened subarachnoid space in the posterior fossa between the dorsum of the medulla and the cerebellum. From here it flows into the subarachnoid spaces over the hemisphere and the spinal subarachnoid space for resorption.

RESORPTION OF CSF

Resorption occurs by two processes. Its water diffuses back into the blood through the walls of small blood vessels. Electrolytes and other components are resorbed by metabolic processes through ventricular walls and through arachnoid villi (Figure 30). Villi are numerous along the superior sagittal sinus, in basal cisterns, and along spinal nerve roots.

In persons beyond middle age, masses of connective tissue deposit over arachnoid villi. These form lumps readily visible to the naked eye — arachnoid granulations. They appear of no clinical significance, as they do not prevent adequate resorption of CSF.

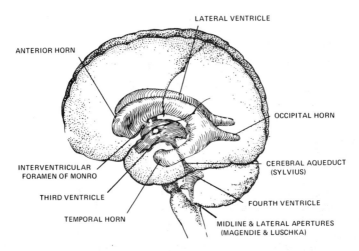

FIGURE 27. The ventricular system. (Reproduced, with permission, from Chusid: *Correlative Neuroanatomy & Functional Neurology, 15th ed.* Lange Medical Publications.)

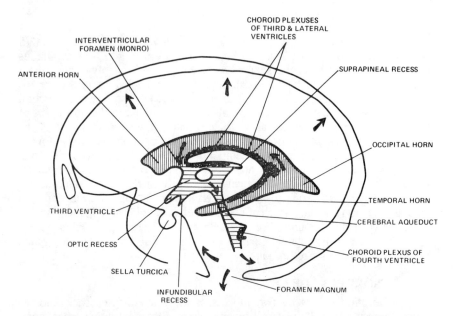

FIGURE 28. Lateral view of ventricular system with choroids plexuses. Arrows indicate directions of CSF flow, for eventual resorption into the superior sagittal sinus or into lymph channels about spinal nerves.

CISTERNS

In several regions called cisterns, the subarachnoid spaces are widened. These cisterns are usually named by their location: cisterna magna (cerebello-medullaris), chiasmatic cistern, interpeduncular cistern, pontine cistern, superior cistern.

CSF may take part in certain metabolic functions, but its major known function is buoyancy, protecting the brain against mechanical shocks.

Hydrocephalus (water on the brain) refers to an abnormally increased volume of CSF. This may result from blockage of CSF circulation, or from the prenatal or postnatal destruction of brain tissue, replaced by CSF.

In communicating hydrocephalus, the passage of CSF from ventricles to subarachnoid spaces is free. Noncommunicating hydrocephalus is present when this flow is blocked.

THE DURA

Surrounding the arachnoid and lying directly against it with only a moist potential space interposed, the dura (Latin = hard) is the third meningeal layer, a thick and very strong sheet of connective tissue. As it is the outermost meningeal layer, the dura fuses with the periosteum inside the skull to form a single layer in the adult. The meninges form dural root sheaths around each cranial and spinal nerve (Figure 6). Their connective tissue continues peripherally without interruption as the epineureum and perineureum of the peripheral nerves.

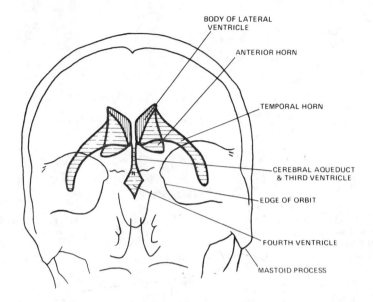

BODY OF LATERAL VENTRICLE

ANTERIOR HORN

TEMPORAL HORN

CEREBRAL AQUEDUCT & THIRD VENTRICLE

EDGE OF ORBIT

FOURTH VENTRICLE

MASTOID PROCESS

FIGURE 29. Anteroposterior view of the ventricular system, as seen in a ventriculogram.

Two major folds of dura within the cranial cavity divide it into compartments. The midline falx (cerebri) (Figures 30, 31) is a sickle-shaped (falx = sickle) double sheet of dura separating the two cerebral hemispheres and attached to the cranial vault along the midline superior sagittal sinus. Right and left leaves of the tentorium (cerebelli) form a tent-like roof over the cerebellum in the posterior fossa, separating the cerebellum from the occipital lobe of the cerebrum. It divides the cranial cavity into infratentorial and supratentorial compartments, the former containing cerebellum and brain stem, the latter the cerebral hemispheres.

LUMBAR PUNCTURE

Occasionally, need exists to examine CSF for diagnostic purposes, or to inject therapeutic agents or anesthetics into the subarachnoid spaces. Since these spaces surround the entire CNS, theoretically CSF might be obtained anywhere. Caudally, however, the spinal cord extends only to the second lumbar level (L2), while the subarachnoid space extends further, to second and third sacral level (S2-3) (Figures 6 and 7). Therefore, the lumbar puncture needle is inserted at L5-S1 or L4-5, to enter the CSF space without danger to the spinal cord.

CLINICAL EXAMPLE 2

A patient came to the emergency room with high fever, complaining of a severe headache and stiff neck. Meningitis was suspected so a lumbar puncture was performed. List the layers pierced in inserting the LP needle into the lumbar subarachnoid space.

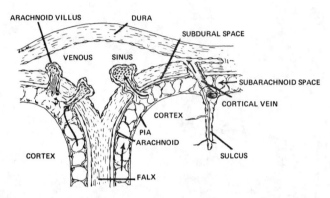

FIGURE 30. Relations of pia-arachnoid, arachnoid villi, and cortical veins to dural sinuses. Arrows indicate CSF or blood flow. (Reproduced, with permission, from Spurling: *Practical Neurological Diagnosis, 4th ed.* Charles C. Thomas, Springfield, IL, 1950.)

Discussion

After appropriate antisepsis, the LP needle is inserted through the skin at the space between L4 and L5 or between L5 and S1 spinous processes. The needle passes through subcutaneous fatty tissue into paraspinous muscle or the fascia surrounding the muscle. Then the advancing needle 'pops' as it pierces the ligamentum flavum between the vertebral laminae (see Figure 7). After a few millimeters of epidural space, the needle 'pops' again as it pierces the dura, usually simultaneously piercing the filmy arachnoid to enter the subarachnoid space around the cauda equina (see Figure 6). CSF is then removed for study.

If the patient does have meningitis, there will be an increased number of cells in the CSF, usually polymorphonuclear white cells (review Table 5).

CLINICAL EXAMPLE 3

A boy, 9 years old, came to the neurosurgery clinic with a brain tumor (medulloblastoma) of the fourth ventricle. X-ray therapy caused temporary regression of the tumor, but it eventually grew large enough to fill the ventricle and block the flow of CSF. The child then developed acute hydrocephalus. Which parts of the ventricular system enlarged?

Discussion

See Figure 28. The block of CSF flow in the fourth ventricle will result in hydrocephalic enlargement of all ventricular spaces 'upstream': the cerebral aqueduct, the third ventricle, and both lateral ventricles.

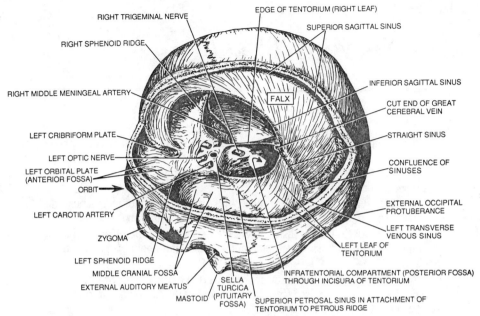

FIGURE 31. Interior of the skull with retained dural folds and other important structures.

CLINICAL EXAMPLE 4

A 27-year-old farm worker from the southern San Joaquin Valley of California became ill with progressively increasing headache, stiff neck, variable fever, and eventually increasing stupor. Suspecting coccidioidal meningitis (Valley Fever) a lumbar puncture was done. Discuss the findings.

Discussion

Spinal fluid pressure was slightly increased (200 mm H_2O), cell count was 175 lymphocytes per mm^2, protein was 75 mg/dl, and glucose was 10 mg/dl. All these variants from the normal (refer to Table 5) confirm the presence of a chronic meningitis, such as caused by coccidioides or tuberculosis. With an acute meningitis, such as caused by meningococcus or a variety of other bacteria, the excess cell count would have been polymorphonuclear leucocytes (note Clinical Example 2). Increased protein and decreased glucose occur in many kinds of meningitis.

STUDY QUESTIONS

1. Sketch the human ventricular system, with labels.
2. Why is a lumbar puncture done at the L4-5 or L5-S1 level?
3. What is meant by hydrocephalus?
4. What is the choroid plexus? What is its function?
5. Where are the subarachnoid spaces?
6. What are the basal cisterns?
7. Describe the circulation of CSF.

5 Nervous Tissue

Three main cellular components make up the mammalian central nervous system:

1. Neurons or nerve cells, the primary functioning units, constituting 50-60 percent of the mass of the brain.

2. Glia (Greek = glue) or neuroglia, which provide mechanical and metabolic support, and make up 30-50 percent of the brain's mass.

3. Vascular tissues: walls of arteries, arterioles, capillaries and veins, the blood inside them, and associated elements. These total about 10 percent of the brain's mass.

In addition to these three formed tissues, the extracellular or intercellular interstitial spaces contain extracellular fluid and colloidal matrix amounting to 5-10 percent of the mass of the brain.

These figures vary from region to region within the brain, and increase and decrease with neuronal activity. For example, local blood flow increases strikingly in physiologically active areas of cortex, as in the visual cortex during vision, or in epileptic cortex during a seizure.

NEUROGLIA

Two distinct ectodermal cell lines develop in the early neural tube of vertebrates: spongioblasts and neuroblasts. The former develop into the various types of neuroglia, the latter become neurons.

In the adult, four types of neuroglia have been identified: (1) ependyma; (2) astrocytes or astroglia; (3) oligodendrocytes or oligodendroglia; (4) microglia. Three derive from ectodermal spongioblasts. The fourth, microglia, are mesodermal derivatives, brought into the CNS with ingrowing embryonic blood vessels.

Primitive ependymal cells line the embryonic neural tube, where they divide to form all CNS cells, neuronal and glial. In the adult, specialized ciliated ependymal cells line the ventricles. As mentioned earlier, ependymal cells are not joined by tight junctions, and so allow free percolation of CSF from the ventricular cavities into the extracellular spaces of the brain parenchyma. This free movement of CSF is important in maintaining the electrolyte concentrations around the neurons of the CNS. Astrocytes are star-shaped cells (astro = star) of two types. Fibrous astrocytes, found predominantly in fiber tracts of the CNS, contain heavy bands of specific fibrils for mechanical support. Protoplasmic astrocytes contain fewer fibrils, and predominate in nuclei or cortex, i.e., in neuronal collections. Astrocyte processes form a subpial layer of tissue on the surface of the CNS, and may act there in molecular transport. Astrocytes throughout the CNS act as potassium 'sinks,' removing K^+ from the extraneuronal fluid to maintain the electrolyte concentration necessary for normal neuronal function.

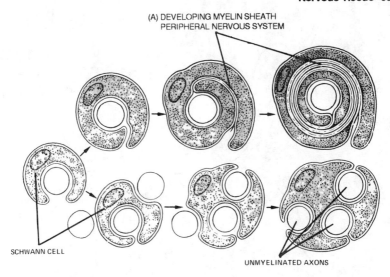

(A) DEVELOPING MYELIN SHEATH
PERIPHERAL NERVOUS SYSTEM

SCHWANN CELL

UNMYELINATED AXONS

(B) ELECTRON MICROGRAPH RECONSTRUCTION
MYELIN IN CENTRAL NERVOUS SYSTEM

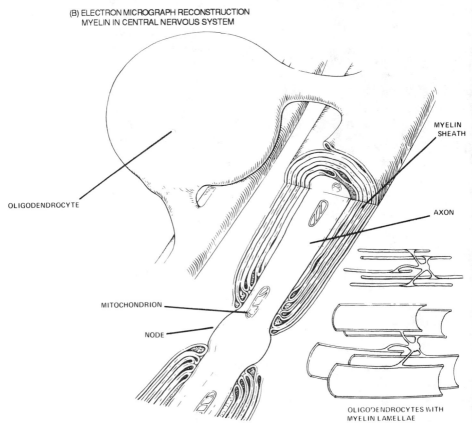

MYELIN
SHEATH

OLIGODENDROCYTE

AXON

MITOCHONDRION

NODE

OLIGODENDROCYTES WITH
MYELIN LAMELLAE

FIGURE 32. Myelination in peripheral nerve (A) and in central nervous system (B).

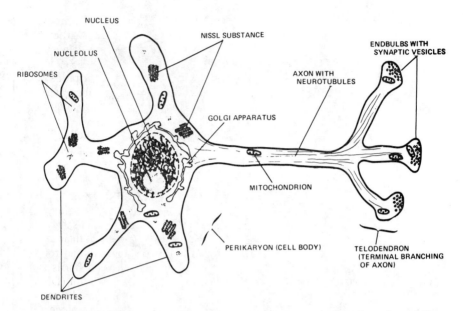

FIGURE 33. Neuron with examples of various cellular organelles. Actual numbers of these organelles are much greater than shown here.

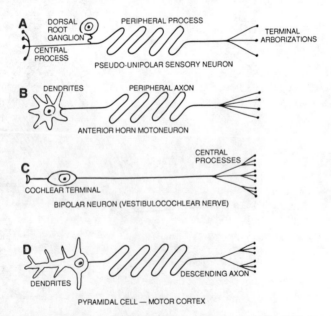

FIGURE 34. Several types of neurons in the mammalian nervous system. The 'folded' axons suggest the great length of these processes. Many neurons, particularly 'interneurons' have much shorter axons, and some have no axon at all.

Brain capillaries are encased in 'astrocytic feet,' expansions of astrocytic processes forming part of the blood-brain barrier (Chapter 3). Astrocytes, particularly of fibrous type, multiply rapidly by mitosis following damage to nervous tissue to form glial scars or gliosis.

Oligodendroglia (oligo = few; dendro = branch) possess fewer processes than astrocytes. They produce myelin sheaths surrounding nerve fibers within the CNS (Figure 32), and have the potential for changing into macrophages to engulf degenerating neurons.

Microglia (micro = small) are smaller than the other glia cells. They derive from nonnervous, mesodermal primordia and also have the capability to act as macrophages.

NEURONS

All neurons derive from embryonic ectoderm. They possess organelles and morphologic and metabolic characteristics of most animal cells (Figure 33). Their triple external membrane consists mostly of lipoproteins, their cytoplasm contains mitochondria, Golgi apparatus, lysosomes, smooth and rough endoplasmic reticulum (RER = Nissl's substance), ribosomes, and fibrils and tubules (neurofibrils, neurotubules). Their nucleus contains chromatin (DNA) and a prominent nucleolus (RNA), and is bounded by a perforated nuclear envelope. Neurons vary from 5 to 100 microns in diameter, and have processes of widely varying complexity and length, from a few microns to a meter or more. See Figure 34 for examples of several neuronal types.

Neurons have no mitotic capability. Once destroyed, they cannot be replaced by mitosis of other cells. Neuronal division ceases about age 6 months. At that age we have the largest number of neurons we will ever have.

It would be useful to review at this time the functions of various cellular organelles in a textbook of histology or cellular physiology.

SPECIAL CHARACTERISTICS OF NEURONS

For the reception of incoming nerve impulses, neurons have branching processes called dendrites. They vary greatly in complexity and length. Axons, which carry nerve impulses away from the neuronal cell body (soma or perikaryon), also vary in complexity but are usually longer than dendrites. Axons, commonly called nerve fibers, have diameters from 0.1 to 20 microns. They may be covered by an interrupted myelin sheath of fatty material, or, more often, are unmyelinated (review Figure 32). Axons affect other neurons through specialized terminals called synapses.

CLASSIFICATION OF NEURONS

Neurons are commonly classified in various ways, depending on the context. These classifications are, of course, not mutually exclusive, nor do they exhaust the possibilities:

1. Morphology. This is suggested by Figure 34.

2. Function. Each neuron can be classified by the function it mediates in the intact organism.

3. Chemically. This refers most often to neurotransmitters, the chemical substances which act on other neurons at their synaptic junctions.

4. Location. Ordinarily defined by position of the cell body in specific central nuclei or specific peripheral ganglia.

CONVERGENCE AND DIVERGENCE

Most neurons receive hundreds or thousands of converging synaptic connections from other neurons. Moreover, axons often branch profusely to terminate in synapses on many other neurons. These effect the neurophysiologic processes of convergence and divergence (Figure 35). Dendrites also often branch exuberantly, increasing further the possibilities for convergence of incoming impulses. Figure 36 depicts examples of axonal branching (divergence) and dendritic branching (convergence) in the human spinal cord.

AXOPLASMIC FLOW = AXON TRANSPORT

Axons or dendrites may extend 1 meter from the perikaryon, with total volumes as great as 100 times that of the perikaryon, and surface areas 1000 times as great. These elongated fibers require proteins and other substances produced in the perikaryon. To reach the processes where they are needed, these substances flow in the cytoplasm away from the cell body by energy (i.e., ATP) -dependent processes in at least two components, at 1-4 mm/day, and at 100-400 mm/day, called slow and fast axoplasmic flow. Neurotubules are believed to carry out part of the axoplasmic transport, inasmuch as the drug colchicine, which depolymerizes neurotubules, prevents fast axoplasmic flow.

Whether newly developing in the embryo, or regenerating after injury, the maximum rate of growth of nerve fibers is about 1 mm/day, similar to the velocity of slow axoplasmic flow, suggesting possible connection between slow axoplasmic flow and fiber growth.

Because of dependence on materials from the cell body, a cut axon degenerates, with a histological sequence called Wallerian degeneration (Figure 37). Historically, Wallerian degeneration argued strongly in favor of the neuron

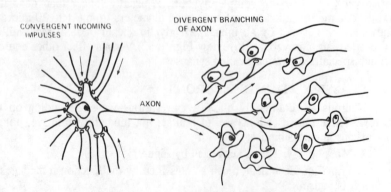

FIGURE 35. Convergence of impulses onto the neuron on the left; divergence of impulses from that neuron onto the neurons at the right.

doctrine, i.e., that each neuron is an individual cell, and not part of a cytoplasmic syncytium.

Axoplasmic flow also occurs toward the cell body, at about 100 mm/day. A peripheral injury, such as the lesion of Figure 37, sends chemical agents toward the cell body which trigger the change called chromatolysis. The Nissl substance (RER = rough endoplasmic reticulum) breaks up and moves to the periphery of the cell, the nucleus becomes eccentric, and the perikaryon swells.

DYNAMIC POLARITY

A nerve impulse travels along the axon and activates the synapse (Figure 35), causing secretion of chemical neurotransmitter from the synaptic vesicles in the end-bulb (Figure 33). The neurotransmitter diffuses onto the membrane of the next neuron and induces there a new potential. Because only the presynaptic side of the synapse contains neurotransmitter, chemical synapses can act only in one direction. Under the electron microcope this is made evident by the presence of neurotransmitter-containing synaptic vesicles only on one side of each chemical synapse. In the living organism, therefore, nerve action potentials travel toward the cell body along dendritic processes, and away from the cell body along axons. In the laboratory, however, it is easy to demonstrate that the nerve impulse can travel in either direction. The unidirectionality of impulse transmission in the living body depends on the unidirectionality of synaptic function. This concept is called dynamic polarity.

MEMBRANE POTENTIAL

Cell membranes bound most living cells. As part of the life process, differences in concentration of various ions are maintained between inside and outside of cell membranes. These concentration differences are maintained by the action of protein structures called 'sodium-potassium pumps' or 'sodium-potassium ATPase' which are located in the cell membrane and which use the metabolic energy of ATP to pump sodium out of the cell and potassium in. These metabolically-maintained concentration gradients across the cell membrane provide the source of energy for the electrical potentials observed during neuronal activity. In mammalian neurons, potassium (K^+) concentration differences across the membrane account for most of the resting membrane potential.

Resting membrane potentials of many mammalian neurons fall between 60 and 70 mV, outside positive to the inside (Figure 38). This potential is not truly resting, but is rather metastable, depending on the semipermeability of the cell membrane (i.e., that it is permeable to some ions and not to others) and on the fact that potassium ions diffuse outward cross the cell membrane more easily than sodium ions diffuse inward, making the outside positive with respect to the inside.

To first approximation, the potential can be calculated from concentrations using the Nernst equation for potassium, by using human body temperature and logarithms to the base 10:

$$E_K = 61 \log(K_{out} / K_{in})$$

Similar calculations give the electrical potential expected from the sodium concentration gradient. The actual electrical potential as a work function, however, depends also on the ionic permeability or conductance of the neuronal membrane for various ions, in particular, potassium, sodium, proteins, and in many instances calcium.

The conductance of the neuronal membrane for potassium ions (g_K) is about ten times or more that for sodium (g_{Na}). As a result, potassium ions diffuse down their concentration gradients (i.e., out of the cell) much more readily than sodium (which diffuses in). Negative protein ions within the cell are quite unable to penetrate the membrane (the membrane is semipermeable). so that as the positively-charged potassium ions diffuse out, they leave an equal negative charge (the protein ions) inside the membrane. Because less than one-tenth as much sodium diffuses in as potassium diffuses out, potassium chiefly determines the resting membrane potential.

Although chloride has a conductance (g_{Cl}) about four times that of sodium, it is not involved in determining the resting membrane potential, because it is not pumped across most of the cell membranes we are concerned with. Its concentrations are passively determined by membrane potential.

The permeabilities, or in electrical terms conductances, of the membrane ions are not characteristic of the cell membrane itself, but rather depend on the presence of complex protein structures embedded in the membrane. These protein structures are pierced by pores or 'gates,' through which water, ions, and sometimes other substances can move either inward or outward across the membrane. There are specific gates for potassium, for sodium, for chloride, and in many instances for other ionic or non-ionic substances.

Few potassium ions actually diffuse across the membrane. They charge the outside of the membrane, acting as a very efficient capacitor, in a layer of positivity only about 0.1 micron thick or less. The resting membrane potential is the potential at which the capacitive charge across the membrane causes just as many positive potassium ions to be attracted back into the cell by the internal negativity as are forced to diffuse out by the concentration gradient.

Because of the very small number of ions actually moving across the membrane, the overall concentrations of internal and external ions do not change appreciably.

As hinted above, conductances of the membrane for the various ions need to be included in accurate calculation of membrane potentials. The Goldman equation takes these additional factors into account:

$$E = (g_{Na}E_{Na} + g_K E_K)/(g_{Na} + g_K)$$

(The Goldman equation for resting potential)

TABLE 6. Concentrations of sodium, potassium, and chloride ions

		Human muscle	Cat nerve
Na+	Intracellular	12 mE	18 mEq
	Extracellular	140 mEq	135 mEq
K+	Intracellular	80 mEq	166 mEq
	Extracellular	4.5 mEq	5 mEq
Cl-	Intracellular		4 mEq
	Extracellular (human CSF)	120 mEq	

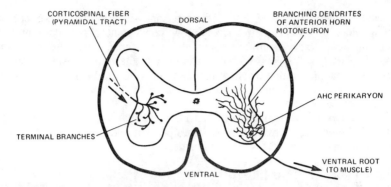

FIGURE 36. Spinal cord cross-section depicting pyramidal tract terminals on the left, and an anterior horn motoneuron (AHC) dendritic tree on the right. AHC dendrites receive synaptic inputs from pyramidal tract axons and many other sources.

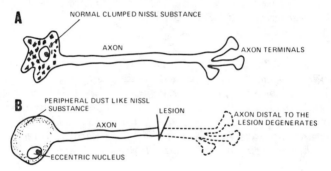

FIGURE 37. (A) Normal neuron. (B) Wallerian degeneration of axon distal to a lesion; chromatolysis of the cell body.

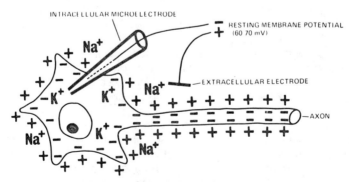

FIGURE 38. Resting membrane potential of a mammalian neuron as measured between an intracellular microelectrode and the extracellular space.

For present purposes, it is less important to perform rigorous computations than to recognize intuitively how conductances and concentration gradients relate to the membrane potential. For example, a decrease in external potassium (K_O) will increase the concentration gradient from inside to outside the cell membrane, with a resultant increase in net outward potassium diffusion and increase in membrane potential. This increase in membrane potential is called hyperpolarization.

Conversely, an increase in external potassium will decrease the concentration gradient, decreasing net outward potassium diffusion and decreasing the membrane potential. This is depolarization.

CLINICAL EXAMPLE 5

A woman, age 50 years, suffered from vomiting and diarrhea for 2 days, presumably as a result of a gastrointestinal infection. When seen, arms and legs were very weak, and she was beginning to experience some difficulty breathing. Treatment to stop the vomiting and antibiotics for the infection made it possible to give her a diet supplemented with potassium chloride, following which her weakness rapidly disappeared.

Discussion

Vomitus contains high concentrations of potassium salts, so that one of the complications of continued vomiting is hypo-kalemia (abnormally low blood potassium). Low blood potassium results in low extracellular potassium, hyperpolarizing neuronal and muscle fiber membranes, so that her muscles could not contract normally. Replacement of the lost potassium corrects the hyperpolarization and contractility returns to normal.

ACTION POTENTIAL

A major function of neurons is the transmission of information in the form of nerve impulses or action potentials, to other neurons, to muscles (where they cause contraction), or to glands (where they cause secretion). The nerve action potential has an electrical amplitude of 100-120 mV, and a duration of about 1 msec. With proper equipment, it can be recorded (Figure 39).

The upward deviation of the action potential on the oscilloscope screen of Figure 39 represents a brief period of negativity of the outside of the axonal membrane relative to the inside, i.e., a depolarization. This electrical event results from an abrupt, large increase in the conductance of the membrane to sodium (g_{Na}), i.e., the sodium gates suddenly open wide. This is associated with a sudden increase in the inward movement of sodium ions, making the inside of the axon positive and outside negative. This external negativity immediately sets up 'local currents' with the adjacent resting membrane's external positivity, as in Figure 40. These local currents depolarize the adjacent membrane, so that the externally negative action potential enters the picture from the left, moving toward the right through the progressive depolarization of successive bits of axonal membrane by the local currents.

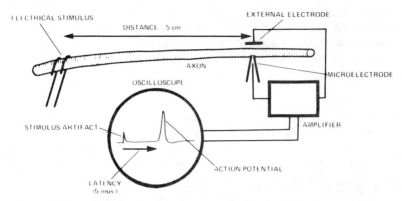

FIGURE 39. Action potential recording from a single axon. Velocity of propagation equals distance divided by latency: V = (5 cm/5 msec) = 10 meters/second.

As the action potential proceeds toward the right, the axonal membrane on the left repolarizes. This results from two changes caused by the depolarization: first, the suddenly-opened sodium gates close, so that sodium ions can no longer enter the cell (g_{Na} decreases), and then potassium gates open (potassium conductance g_K increases) to reconstitute the external positivity. Note the importance of ionic permeabilities in these potential changes. Refer back to the Goldman equation on p. 38.

Velocities of conduction along unmyelinated nerve fibers vary from 0.5 to 2 M/sec. The velocity depends directly on the size of the axon, because the amperage of the local currents, and therefore the rate of depolarization, is inversely proportional to the ohmic resistance of the axoplasm. The larger the axon, the lower its resistance, the greater the local currents, and the faster the velocity of impulse propagation.

MYELINATION

In contrast to the unmyelinated axon of Figure 40, many nerve fibers are covered by an insulating layer of myelin 1-5 microns thick. They are myelinated, in interrupted segments 100-1000 microns long (see Figures 32, 41). Under the electron microscope, myelin is seen to consist of spiral layers of lipoprotein. These layers are the cell membrane of Schwann cells in the peripheral nervous system, and of oligodendroglia in the CNS, wrapped around the axon. Each myelin segment is produced and supported by a single cell (see Figure 32).

SALTATORY CONDUCTION

Normal human peripheral nerves conduct at 40-70 M/sec, exceeding velocities of unmyelinated axons several-fold—Table 7. These faster velocities result directly from the insulating effect of the myelin segments. In Figure 41, the local currents operate just as in unmyelinated axons, but depolarize the axonal membrane only at the nodes, where there is no myelin. Thus, the action potential jumps from node to node, much faster than if the axon were unmyelinated. This mode of propagation is called saltatory conduction (Latin, saltare = jump).

Note that fiber types of similar diameters and velocities have varied functions, and are labeled to correspond to these functions. In mammalian peripheral nerves, the proportions of large myelinated to small myelinated to unmyelinated fibers, is about 1:5:30.

CLINICAL EXAMPLE 6

A lady with long-standing diabetes was referred to the neurology clinic because of numbness and weakness of her hands. On examination, most sensation was lost from both of her hands, and her grip was very weak. Nerve conduction studies showed median and ulnar velocities of 35-40 M/sec rather than the normal 55-65 M/sec.

Discussion

This is the clinical syndrome of diabetic neuropathy. The disease disturbs the metabolism of Schwann cells, often leading to their degeneration and degeneration of the myelin segments supported by them. This pathology is called segmental demyelination.

Velocity of conduction along the demyelinated segments is much slower than normal, because saltatory conduction is not possible. Many motor and sensory axons may die as well, causing weakness and loss of sensation.

ACTION POTENTIAL THRESHOLD

Action potentials are all-or-none phenomena, either occurring to the full extent or not occurring at all. The all-or-none action potential is triggered by potential changes which are not all-or-none, but graded, i.e., varying in amplitude depending on stimulus intensity.

Small voltages applied to the neuron will cause a change in the local membrane potential, but won't trigger an action potential unless the change reaches a threshold value. In the most commonly studied mammalian neuron,

TABLE 7. Classification of peripheral nerve fibers

Diameter (microns)	Velocity (M/sec)	Function	Designation
12-20	70-120	Motor	A-alpha = extrafusal motor A-beta = motor
		Sensory	Ia = spindle afferents Ib = Golgi afferents
5-12	30-70	Motor	A-gamma = intrafusal motor
		Sensory	II = sensory spindle afferents, touch from skin
2-5	12-30	Motor	?
		Sensory	III = pain from muscle, sensation from skin
3	3-15	Motor	B = preganglionic autonomic
Unmyelinated			
0.5-1	0.5-2	Motor	C = postganglionic autonomic
		Sensory	IV = pain

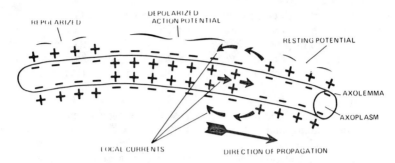

FIGURE 40. Propagation of an action potential along an unmyelinated axon.

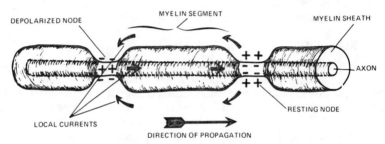

FIGURE 41. Saltatory conduction of an action potential from node to node; myelinated axon

the anterior horn motoneuron (AHC) of the cat, action potential threshold approximates 15 mV depolarization (see Figure 42).

Subthreshold voltage changes cause slight increases in sodium conductance (g_{Na}) through reversible changes in the openness of the sodium gates. At threshold, the sodium gates have opened so widely that the inward flow (flux) of sodium ions exceeds the outward flow of potassium ions, following which the sodium conductance almost instantaneously (time measured in microseconds) increases many-fold. The resultant surge of sodium ions inward across the membrane causes a brief reversal of the membrane potential. The action potential overshoots the zero level, i.e., the membrane becomes externally negative, because g_{Na} temporarily greatly exceeds g_K, and more sodium diffuses in than potassium ions diffuse out.

As implied, potassium conductance (g_K) begins to increase simultaneously with g_{Na}, but more slowly. A little later, the increasing outward movement of potassium ions counteracts the external negativity of the action potential and reconstitutes the resting potential. During this interval, g_{Na} returns spontaneously to its resting level.

Return of g_{Na} and g_K to resting levels prepares the neuronal membrane for the next action potential.

For a millisecond, while the membrane permeabilities (and conductances) are maximum, no further action potential can be evoked. This is called the absolute refractory period. For the next few milliseconds, threshold is higher than the resting level — the relative refractory period.

Two conductance changes cause the absolute refractory period. First, at the peak of the action potential the sodium gates open fully and cannot be opened further; g_{Na} cannot increase beyond that point. Second, the sodium gates immediately begin to close as a result of the depolarization. Note that they open rapidly in response to depolarization, then close, more slowly, in response to the same depolarization. Increase in potassium conductance g_K beyond the resting level, also due to depolarization, gives rise to the relative refractory period, and to the after-hyperpolarization pictured in Figure 42.

Few sodium and potassium ions traverse the membrane to cause the various normal potentials, because they are restricted to a layer very close to the membrane. Thus, no significant changes in concentration can be detected, and the sodium-potassium pump has no difficulty keeping up. Even after inactivation of the pump by drugs such as ouabain or dinitrophenol thousands of action potentials can occur.

These threshold phenomena apply to most of the neuronal membrane.

FUNCTION OF CHEMICAL SYNAPSES

Under the electron microscope, chemical synapses are seen to contain clusters of synaptic vesicles, usually 200-400 angstroms in diameter, in the presynaptic axonal end-bulb. These vesicles contain neurotransmitter, and fuse with the membrane of the end-bulb to release the neurotransmitter into the synaptic cleft if calcium ions are present. See Figures 33 and 43.

When an action potential arrives at the end-bulb, it depolarizes calcium gates in the membrane of the end-bulb, causing them to open (g_{Ca} increases), allowing calcium ions to diffuse into the end-bulb from extracellular spaces. In the presence of Ca^{++} synaptic vesicles fuse with the presynaptic membrane, and open, so that their contained neurotransmitter is released into the synaptic gap. Rapidly diffusing across the gap (200 angstroms = 0.02 microns), the neurotransmitter molecules alter the conductance of the postsynaptic membrane to one or more ions (g_{Na}, g_K, or g_{Cl}), thereby inducing a postsynaptic potential (PSP). The PSP may be excitatory (EPSP) or inhibitory (IPSP). If the EPSP exceeds threshold, an action potential is triggered in the postsynaptic neuron.

These events usually require 0.5 to 1 msec — the synaptic delay.

In addition to synapses between axon terminals and dendrites or cell bodies (axodendritic or axosomatic), synaptic junctions may occur between dendrites (dendrodendritic), between axons (axo-axonal) or from dendrites to axons (dendroaxonal).

ELECTRICAL SYNAPSES

Most mammalian synapses appear to be chemically mediated, but a few examples are known where the synapse functions through direct electrical connection. Such electrical synapses or gap junctions have no synaptic cleft, no synaptic vesicles, and no synaptic delay. Electrical resistance is diminished by pores piercing the fused membranes of the two adjacent cells (Figure 43).

POSTSYNAPTIC POTENTIALS

Arrival of an action potential at a synaptic end-bulb initiates a calcium-mediated process through which synaptic vesicles discharge their neurotransmitter into the synaptic cleft. Excitatory neurotransmitters increase sodium

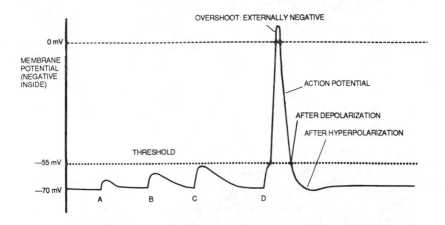

FIGURE 42. Increasing electrical impulses applied to a neuron at A, B, C, and D. At D the applied potential exceeded threshold; triggering an all-or-none action potential.

conductance (g_{Na}) in the postsynaptic membrane, causing depolarization in the form of an excitatory postsynaptic potential (EPSP) — Figure 44. Inhibitory synapses increase postsynaptic conductance of potassium and/or chloride ions (g_K, g_{Cl}). Increased g_K hyperpolarizes the membrane, making excitation more difficult: i.e., depolarization is inhibited. Increased g_{Cl} does not change the membrane potential significantly, but increased mobility of negative chloride ions tends to short out depolarizing EPSPs, also accomplishing an inhibitory effect (see Figures 44 and 46C).

A neuron may produce more than one neurotransmitter, contrary to a long-held hypothesis. Exactly how these multiple neurotransmitters operate is now being investigated. For present purposes, it will be appropriate to treat each synapse as functioning with a single neurotransmitter. Even with a single neurotransmitter, different postsynaptic effects may be seen at different synapses because the protein 'receptors' in the postsynaptic membrane of the synapses differ widely, each reacting with its neurotransmitter in a specific way. Some increase sodium conductance, some potassium conductance, some chloride conductance, or they may cause effects on other ions, even including decreasing conductances of specific ions.

As mentioned earlier, chemical synapses operate in one direction, from the axonal end-bulb toward the postsynaptic neuron, because synaptic vesicles containing neurotransmitter occur only in the presynaptic end-bulb.

MINIATURE POSTSYNAPTIC POTENTIALS (MPSP)

Even at rest, very small PSPs with amplitudes 0.1 to 1 mV, and durations less than 1 msec are observed in most synapses. They occur randomly, and are the electrical evidence of the random discharge of one or a small number of synaptic vesicles into the synaptic cleft. Full-sized EPSPs or IPSPs result from the simultaneous discharge of about 100 synaptic vesicles, induced by an incoming action potential.

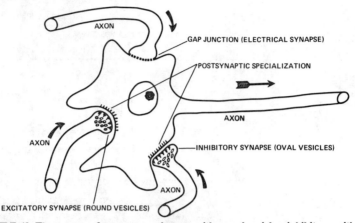

FIGURE 43. Three types of synapses: excitatory, with round vesicles; inhibitory, with oval or flat vesicles; electrical, without vesicles. Arrows indicate direction of action potential propagation.

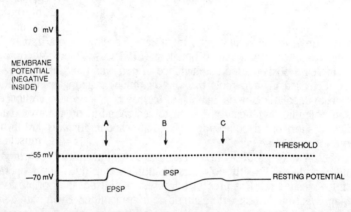

FIGURE 44. (A) Amplitude of EPSP depolarization is around 5 mV. (B) Amplitude of IPSP hyperpolarization is around 4 mV. (C) Chloride inhibitory synapses cause little change in membrane potential.

CLINICAL EXAMPLE 7

A standard neurophysiological procedure applied to patients is the 'H reflex.' Electrical stimulation of the tibial nerve at the knee induces reflex contraction of the soleus muscle of the calf which is recordable. If the normal sensory and motor velocities in the reflex path are both 40 M/sec, and the distance from the knee to S1 spinal cord segment is 60 cm, what delay would you expect between stimulation and response?

Discussion

Delay equals distance divided by velocity:

$$T = \frac{D}{V} = \frac{60 \text{ cm} + 60 \text{ cm}}{40 \text{ M/sec}} = 30 \text{ msec}$$

Add to this 1 msec synaptic delay in the spinal cord, gives a total expected delay of 31 msec.

EXCITATION, INHIBITION, SUMMATION

In most instances, a single excitatory postsynaptic potential (EPSP) is insufficient to depolarize the postsynaptic membrane beyond threshold. Several EPSPs must appear simultaneously to summate, depolarize the membrane past threshold, and trigger an action potential (see Figure 45).

In the spinal cord of mammals, EPSPs and IPSPs last 10-20 msec with a rapid rise and slower fall-off. In some situations, durations may be as long as 100 msec.

When an EPSP and an IPSP occur at the same time, they cancel, as graphed in Figure 46A. An IPSP may prevent the achieving of threshold depolarization by summated EPSPs (Figure 46B). Similarly, a chloride inhibitory synapse may prevent summated EPSPs from reaching threshold (Figure 46C).

Most neurons receive many converging synaptic inputs, both excitatory and inhibitory (see Figure 35). An action potential can be triggered only if the excess of EPSPs over IPSPs is sufficient at that instant. Multiple summation is a basic process of mammalian nervous systems. Anterior horn motoneurons (AHC) of the spinal cord are an extensively studied example of this balance between EPSPs and IPSPs. Each AHC receives 5000 to 10,000 synaptic terminals. An action potential develops in the AHC, causing muscle contraction, only if incoming excitatory activity sufficiently exceeds incoming inhibitory activity.

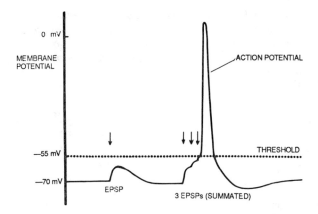

FIGURE 45. A single EPSP produces subthreshold depolarization. Three nearly simultaneous EPSPs summate to exceed threshold and trigger an action potential.

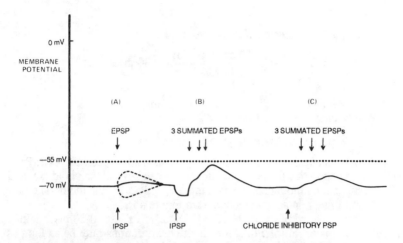

FIGURE 46. (A) Simultaneous EPSP and IPSP cancel. (B) An IPSP prevents three summated EPSPs from depolarizing beyond threshold (compare Figure 45). (C) By shorting out (clamping) the potential, a chloride inhibitory PSP also prevents three summated EPSPs from depolarizing to threshold.

CLINICAL EXAMPLE 8

Certain South American indians use a vegetable extract containing curare as arrow-tip poison in hunting. Curare competes with excitatory neurotransmitter acetylcholine (ACh) for ACh receptors on the postsynaptic membrane of the neuromyal synapse (motor end plate) between motor nerve axon terminals and muscle fibers. How does this kill a monkey pierced by such an arrow?

Discussion

The curare prevents the excitatory effect of ACh on muscle fibers, thus preventing normal contraction of muscles in response to incoming nerve action potentials by competitive inhibition. Paralysis ensues, and the monkey falls out of the tree because it can no longer hang on. It dies because it cannot breathe.

PRESYNAPTIC INHIBITION

A presynaptic inhibitory axon terminal ends in relation to the pre-synaptic end-bulb of an excitatory synapse — it is an axoaxonal synapse (see Figure 47). An action potential arriving at the presynaptic inhibitory terminal discharges neurotransmitter onto the excitatory end-bulb and prevents the latter from discharging its excitatory neurotransmitter onto the postsynaptic neuron. The inhibitory neurotransmitter is usually GABA (gamma amino butyric acid), and acts by increasing chloride conductance, thus shorting out the incoming action potential. It thereby decreases the effectiveness of the excitatory synapse, without directly affecting the postsynaptic neuron at all. Presynaptic inhibition tapers off over a duration of about 100 msec, as shown in Figure 48.

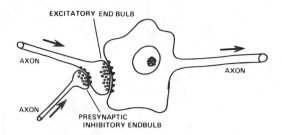

FIGURE 47. Presynaptic inhibition — the presynaptic end-bulb makes axoaxonal synaptic contact with an excitatory terminal rather than with a dendrite or neuronal soma.

SLOW POSTSYNAPTIC POTENTIALS

In a number of locations, synaptic effects have been observed which last much longer — up to several seconds. These may utilize the same neurotransmitters as faster responses (e.g., ACh, dopamine, and possibly others), but are believed to do so through the intermediary of cyclic AMP or cyclic GMP, which alter membrane conductance or the sodium pump over longer periods of time. In addition to the relatively well-understood neurotransmitters listed in Table 8, many other simple neurotransmitters are known, such as aspartic acid, taurine, substance P, and adrenalin (epinephrine). Moreover, in recent years dozens of hormones and hormone-like peptides have been shown to have neurotransmitter actions in a variety of situations. Many of these peptide neurotransmitters appear in the same synapses as the simpler neurotransmitters of Table 8, and may have longer-lasting effects, or even quite different effects on the postsynaptic cell. Understanding neurotransmitter function is basic to understanding nervous system function, and is the basis of much of pharmacology. A large proportion of toxins and commonly-used drugs act primarily on synapses, accentuating or blocking neurotransmitter actions.

GEOGRAPHIC CHARACTERISTICS OF SYNAPTIC ACTIVITY

A short segment of axonal membrane at the axon's attachment to the cell body has the lowest action potential threshold: 15 mV for the AHC, compared to 25 mV for the membrane of the soma. Because of this low threshold, action potentials usually begin here, for which reason it is called the initial segment (IS). Anatomically, the same general region is called the axon hillock. Its cytoplasm contains no Nissl substance (RER), and when examined with the electron microscope, the cell membrane is seen to have a dense undercoating.

An action potential initiated in the initial segment propagates in both directions: outward along the axon, and backward onto the neuronal soma.

Dendrites in most neurons seem unable to sustain a propagated action potential. For this reason, IPSPs or EPSPs applied to dendrites usually have only electrotonic, passive electrical effects on the initial segment. Synapses lying close to the initial segment generally have more effect on the initial segment than synapses farther away. In many neurons, inhibitory synapses predominate on the soma, next to the initial segment -- which gives the neuron an inhibitory bias.

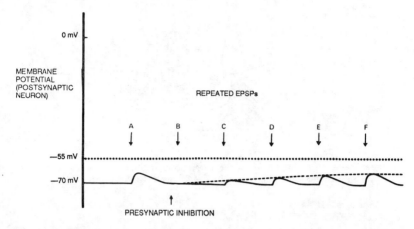

FIGURE 48. Effect of presynaptic inhibition on successive EPSPs, 20 msec apart. A = control EPSP. Note the suppressed EPSP, B, immediately after the presynaptic input, and the gradually increasing EPSP amplitudes. By F, the inhibitory effect has worn off, and the EPSP returns to full amplitude.

RECIPROCAL SYNAPSES

Synapses occur in many types of situations, not solely between axon terminals and dendrites. The reciprocal synapse exemplifies this variability. Here two neurons interact through two adjacent synapses, so that Neuron A excites neuron B through an excitatory synapse (EPSP), then neuron B, through an immediately adjacent synapse, inhibits neuron A (IPSP).

TABLE 8. Mammalian neurotransmitters and their actions

Name	Where found	Action
Acetylcholine (ACh)`	Anterior horn motoneuron	Excitation
	Cortex	Excitation or inhibition
	SNS preganglionic; PSNS	Excitation
Dopamine	Basal ganglia	Inhibition
	Hypothalamus	Prolactin secretion
	Limbic system	Inhibition
	SNS ganglia	Inhibition
Gamma aminobutyric acid (GABA)	CNS	Presynaptic or postsynaptic inhibiltion
Glutamic acid	Cerebellum mossy fibers	Excitation
	Ia spindle afferents	Excitation
Glycine	Spinal cord	Postsynaptic inhibition
Norepinephrine (NE Noradrenalin)	Locus ceruleus	Inhibition
	SNS postganglionic	Excitation
Serotonin (5-hydroxy-tryptamine; 5-HT)	Reticulospinal	Excitation
	Raphe nuclei	Excitation
Endorphins	Periaqueductal gray	Excitation

SNS = sympathetic nervous system
PSNS = parasympathetic nervous system

CLINICAL EXAMPLE 9

A man was brought to the emergency room after attempting suicide with strychnine. He began to convulse, and it was only by dint of deep sedation, artificial respiration, gastric lavage, and muscle relaxants that he survived. Strychnine prevents glycine-induced postsynaptic inhibition (Table 8). How does this cause convulsions?

Discussion

Inhibition is overwhelmingly important in the normal function of the brain. Most systems in the brain consist of converging and diverging sequences of hundreds or thousands of interconnected neurons. If all synapses were excitatory, every incoming impulse would avalanche to all neurons, including motor neurons. Therefore, a large proportion of synapses must be inhibitory. Strychnine inactivates many of the inhibitory synapses of the spinal cord, so that every incoming impulse rapidly spreads to all areas, and convulsive muscle contraction results.

STUDY QUESTIONS

1. Describe the origin of the resting membrane potential.
2. How can it be increased? Decreased?
3. What is the range of velocity of nerve conduction in humans?
4. What variables determine these velocities?
5. What is meant by depolarization of neuronal membranes?
6. What is myelin? Its function? How is it produced?
7. What are Wallerian degeneration and chromatolysis?
8. What is meant by saltatory conduction?
9. Account for the unidirectionality of synaptic function, and for dynamic polarity.
10. Describe four mechanisms by which neuronal activity may be inhibited.
11. What is meant by convergence and by divergence of neuronal impulses?
12. How many synaptic connections does an 'average' mammalian neuron possess? Incoming? Outgoing?
13. What are the functions of various types of neuroglia?
14. Why are inhibitory synapses so important to nervous system function?

6 Somatic Motor Systems

PYRAMIDAL TRACT

From the medical point of view, the pyramidal tract is the most important system of nerve fibers in the CNS, carrying a large portion of the voluntary motor output from the cerebral cortex. Almost all disturbances of voluntary motor function involve the pyramidal tract directly or indirectly. For these reasons, it is often called the upper motor neuron (UMN).

Each pyramidal tract consists of over one million nerve fibers, whose cell bodies lie in the cerebral cortex (areas 4, 6, and 3-1-2 of Brodmann) -- see Figures 50, 51, 52. Some fibers (corticobulbar tracts) descend to cranial nerve nuclei, others (corticospinal tracts) to motor centers of the spinal cord, and yet others to sensory dorsal column nuclei (gracilis and cuneatus) of the medulla, and to sensory dorsal horn neurons in the spinal cord.

The pyramidal tract begins in the cortex (Figures 49 and 50A), descends through the white matter of the cerebrum (the corona radiata — Figure 49), to become concentrated in a bundle in the posterior limb of the internal capsule between the posterior part of the lentiform nucleus and the thalamus (Figure 50B). It then enters the middle third of the cerebral peduncle (Figure 50C), passes through the depths of the pons (Figure 50D) and becomes the pyramid on the ventral face of the medulla (Figures 4 and 50E, see also Figures 74-79). Its name, pyramidal tract, is derived from the pyramids of the medulla, which were anatomically defined long before the tract itself was recognized. At the foramen magnum most of the fibers (80-90%) decussate to form the lateral corticospinal tract (see Figures 4, 49, 50E-F, and 74).

PYRAMIDAL TRACT CONTROL OF LOWER MOTONEURONS

Patterns of termination of motor pyramidal tract (UMN) fibers are sketched in Figures 36, 53, and 54. They may connect monosynaptically with anterior horn motoneurons (AHC) in the cord, or the equivalent in motor cranial nerve nuclei (e.g., facial nucleus, Figure 49) and with many cord and brain stem interneurons (Figure 54) which relay polysynaptically to AHC.

Figure 51 outlines the basic pattern of connections from motor cortex to somatic muscle. The pathway includes a minimum of three cells: the pyramidal tract neuron in the cortex, the anterior horn motoneuron, and the muscle fiber. Two excitatory synapses connect them. This illustration, however, depicts accurately only the large pyramidal tract fibers that directly (monosynaptically) induce voluntary muscle contraction.

These large axons arise from large pyramidal-shaped neurons including the giant cells of Betz in the precentral motor cortex (area 4; see Figures 50A, 51, 52, and 116). They act on muscles of hands, feet, and face which perform delicate movements. The remaining fine fibers in each tract arise from smaller neurons of areas 6 and 3-1-2 as well as 4, and act on inhibitory and excitatory interneurons, to mediate gross motor activity.

Fibers of the pyramidal tract terminate in branching axons distributed diffusely in the transverse plane as in Figures 36 and 53 over several spinal cord segments, corresponding to the individual muscle to be activated. As mentioned above, most of the fibers do not end directly on AHC, but on interneurons within the gray matter of the cord, in the posterior as well as anterior horns. These interneurons often have inhibitory actions, and set up the types of excitatory-inhibitory interactions on AHC referred to on pages 46-48.

Pyramidal tract fibers from the somato-sensory cortex (areas 3-1-2) indirectly affect motor function by inhibiting dorsal column neurons which

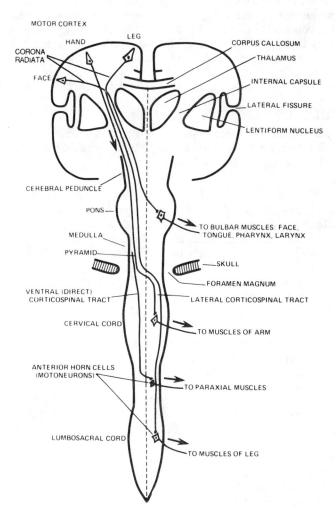

FIGURE 49. Pyramidal tract in outline. Note the inverted cortical face-hand-leg areas, and the crossing (decussation) of 80-90 percent of the fibers at the foramen magnum (see also Figure 52).

relay sensory information from joints and muscles. This probably occurs during rapid movements which are too fast to be corrected by peripheral sensory feedback.

OTHER DESCENDING MOTOR PATHWAYS

The rubrospinal tracts from red nuclei of the midbrain and reticulospinal tracts from reticular nuclei of pons and medulla mediate many aspects of motor function, under volitional control by corticorubral and corticoreticular pathways from the motor cortex. Spasticity (hyperactive muscle stretch reflexes) of upper motor neuron (UMN) lesions probably results mostly from damage to reticulospinal fibers at the same time as pyramidal damage. Paralysis, i.e., loss of volitional motor control, consists of two parts. Lesions of pyramidal tract fibers cause paralysis of fine and delicate movements of fingers, toes, and face, with only weakness (paresis) of other limb movements. Damage to the other motor pathways may cause severe global weakness or paralysis of arms and legs. Clinical lesions often involve all these systems simultaneously, so that vaious mixtures of weakness, spasticity, and sometimes flaccidity are usual.

CLINICAL EXAMPLE 10

A man suffered a stroke, following which he demonstrated inability to use his right hand in manipulative tasks like writing, buttoning his shirt, etc. Where was the lesion?

Discussion

Digital paralysis on the right side points to a lesion of the pyramidal tract; on the right side if it is below the decussation, on the left side if above. Because the only loss was of manipulative abilities, the lesion was most likely restricted to the left pyramid in the medulla (above the decussation) or to a small portion of the primary motor cortex, Area 4. Larger lesions would have caused paralysis of other parts — perhaps the whole extremity, or both arm and leg, or muscles of the face.

VOLITIONAL MOTOR FUNCTION

As an example of the complexity of volitional motor activity, contraction of the biceps muscle may be considered. It results from synaptic excitation of AHC at C5 and C6 levels. Contraction is almost always accompanied by relaxation of the triceps muscle C7 and C8. Thus, the patterned volley of descending UMN impulses simultaneously excites and inhibits AHC at different spinal cord levels. Inhibition always acts through interneurons; excitation may be direct (monosynaptic) or through interneurons. Note also that biceps contraction is usually associated with tightening of shoulder girdle muscles, and neck muscles may be contracted or relaxed. This apparently simple motor event requires synergy (working together) of excitatory and inhibitory synaptic processes from the 11th cranial nerve to upper thoracic levels.

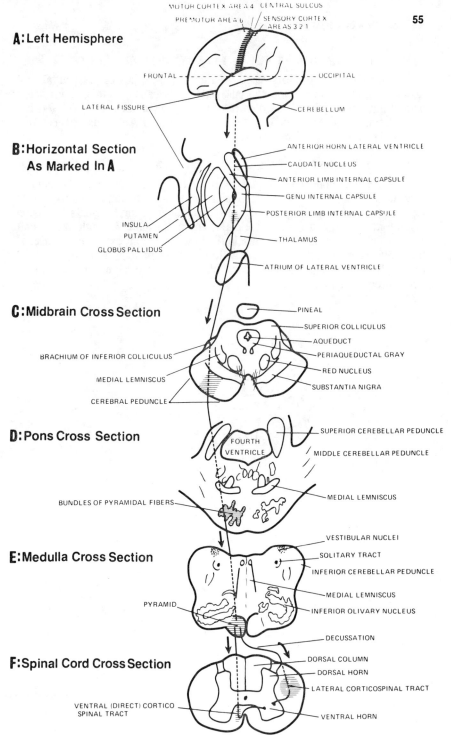

A: Left Hemisphere

MOTOR CORTEX AREA 4 CENTRAL SULCUS
PREMOTOR AREA 6   SENSORY CORTEX
AREAS 3 2 1

FRONTAL — OCCIPITAL

LATERAL FISSURE

CEREBELLUM

B: Horizontal Section
As Marked In **A**

ANTERIOR HORN LATERAL VENTRICLE
CAUDATE NUCLEUS
ANTERIOR LIMB INTERNAL CAPSULE
GENU INTERNAL CAPSULE
POSTERIOR LIMB INTERNAL CAPSULE

INSULA
PUTAMEN
GLOBUS PALLIDUS

THALAMUS

ATRIUM OF LATERAL VENTRICLE

C: Midbrain Cross Section

PINEAL
SUPERIOR COLLICULUS
AQUEDUCT
PERIAQUEDUCTAL GRAY
RED NUCLEUS
SUBSTANTIA NIGRA

BRACHIUM OF INFERIOR COLLICULUS

MEDIAL LEMNISCUS

CEREBRAL PEDUNCLE

D: Pons Cross Section

SUPERIOR CEREBELLAR PEDUNCLE
FOURTH VENTRICLE
MIDDLE CEREBELLAR PEDUNCLE

MEDIAL LEMNISCUS

BUNDLES OF PYRAMIDAL FIBERS

E: Medulla Cross Section

VESTIBULAR NUCLEI
SOLITARY TRACT
INFERIOR CEREBELLAR PEDUNCLE
MEDIAL LEMNISCUS
PYRAMID
INFERIOR OLIVARY NUCLEUS

DECUSSATION

F: Spinal Cord Cross Section

DORSAL COLUMN
DORSAL HORN
LATERAL CORTICOSPINAL TRACT

VENTRAL (DIRECT) CORTICO
SPINAL TRACT

VENTRAL HORN

FIGURE 50. Cortical origin of pyramidal tract and its location at various levels, indicated by cross-hatching (compare Figure 49).

ANTERIOR HORN CELL — LOWER MOTOR NEURON

All motor outflow to striated voluntary muscle passes via ventral root axons of anterior horn motoneurons (AHC). Because of this, Sherrington named these fibers the 'final common path.' Upper motor neuron (UMN) has been defined. Lower motor neuron (LMN) refers to AHC, also called final common path from a different point of view.

MOTOR UNIT

An action potential initiated at one AHC passes peripherally along a ventral root and its branches to cause simultaneous contraction of all its muscle fibers. This contraction is the smallest functional and morphologic subdivision of motor activity, and is therefore called the motor unit. A single motor unit may include as few as 5 to 10 muscle fibers in the small extraocular muscles, for very accurate and gentle contraction. It may include as many as 2000 muscle fibers in the gastrocnemius and other large postural muscles, where the major need is strength.

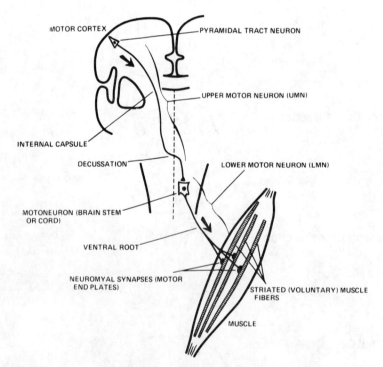

FIGURE 51. Basic two-neuron pattern of motor function, from cortex (UMN) to motoneuron in brain stem or anterior horn of spinal cord.

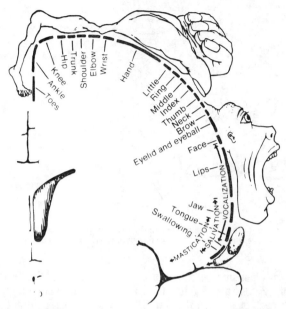

FIGURE 52. Diagram showing the relative size of the parts of the human primary motor cortex from which movements of different parts of the body can be elicited on electrical stimulation. (Reproduced, with permission, from Penfield and Rasmussen: *The Cerebral Cortex of Man*, MacMillan, New York, 1950.)

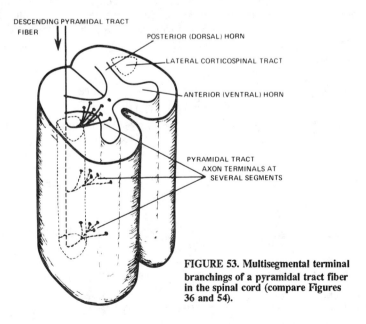

FIGURE 53. Multisegmental terminal branchings of a pyramidal tract fiber in the spinal cord (compare Figures 36 and 54).

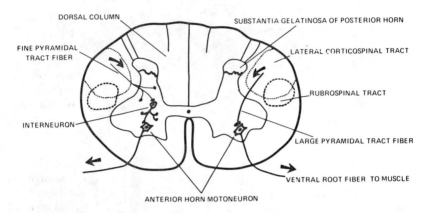

FIGURE 54. Pyramidal tract terminations. Left side: fine fibers mostly end on interneurons. Right side: large fibers end directly on motoneurons. (Correlate with Figures 36, 51, and 53.)

Several mechanisms smooth the contraction of muscles. First, a single motor unit rarely contracts by itself. In all normal movements, many motor units contract, each at its own rhythm. The asynchronous contraction of many motor units at different frequencies smooths the resultant tension (Figure 55). Second, longitudinal elasticity of muscle tissue smooths the tension. Other smoothing mechanisms will be mentioned later.

Strength of contraction of a muscle can be varied over a wide range, by varying the frequency of contraction of individual motor units, and by varying the number of active units.

Both variations occur in response to changes in the overall level of excitability (EPSPs versus IPSPs) of AHC controlling that muscle. These changes may be volitional, resulting from changes in the pattern of descending UMN volleys of action potentials, or may result from reflex changes, some of which will be discussed.

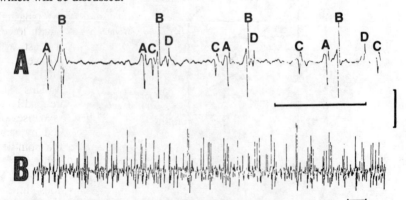

FIGURE 55. (A) Electromyogram (EMG) of gentle contraction of the biceps, obtained with a needle electrode. Individual motor unit action potentials (MUAP) indicated by letters. Note rhythmicity. (B) Same occasion showing interference pattern with slightly stronger contraction. Horizontal scales 100 msec; vertical scale 1 mV.

RECURRENT INHIBITION

Action potentials from AHC result from many types of activation. Uncontrolled activation might lead to continuous repeated action potentials at high frequencies, causing uncontrolled contractions of the motor unit. A built-in inhibitory system prevents this. From each ventral root fiber near its origin a collateral takes off, to synapse with a nearby inhibitory interneuron called a Renshaw cell. The Renshaw cell synapses with many nearby AHC to inhibit their activity. Through this recurrent inhibitory feedback, AHC are prevented from initiating action potentials at frequencies above 50/sec.

MUSCLE STRETCH REFLEX

As a general concept in neural function, a reflex is defined as a process wherein a standard stimulus gives rise to a constant response, through an unvarying neural pathway. Each reflex consists of five functional components: a receptor; an afferent connection; an integrative process; an efferent connection; and an effector. Any of these components may be complex, but in the mammalian nervous system the third, integration within the CNS, is particularly likely to be complex.

Muscle stretch (myotatic) reflexes are stimulated by sudden stretch of neuromuscular spindles in the belly of a muscle (Figures 56 and 57). In the stretch-sensitive primary (annulospiral) endings of the spindle, the stretch generates action potentials which enter the spinal cord via dorsal roots to excite many of the AHC of that muscle, causing its contraction.

In neurological jargon, muscle stretch reflexes are often called 'Deep Tendon Reflexes,' abbreviated DTR.

The knee jerk is a well-known example of the muscle stretch reflex. Tapping the patellar tendon stretches the quadriceps muscle, following which the same muscle contracts reflexly, causing the foot to swing forward. Stretch reflexes can be elicited from most somatic (voluntary) muscles.

Reflex testing gives valuable clues to motor system function (see the 'H' reflex, Clinical Example 7), but appears to be of minor significance in itself. In association with the gamma efferent system, however, it has some important actions.

Clinically, the muscle stretch reflex often becomes more active (spastic) with upper motor neuron (UMN) lesions, and less active (flaccid) with lower motor neuron (LMN) lesions. UMN spasticity results from at least two changes which follow UMN lesions. First, the descending pathways have more inhibitory than excitatory inputs onto anterior horn motoneurons (AHC).

Thus, a UMN lesion decreases inhibitory input to AHC. This disinhibition effectively excites them, and causes them to respond more readily to inputs from the neuromuscular spindle. In addition, as the UMN synapses of AHC degenerate, they leave empty spaces which are reinnervated by new branches from spindle axons. Thus, the synaptic input from the spindles increases, increasing reflex reactivity. It is strongly suspected that other, so far unidentified mechanisms also operate.

'Hyperreflexia,' 'spasticity,' and 'increased DTR' are synonymous clinical terms commonly applied to increased muscle stretch reflexes. Often associated with the increased myotatic reflexes is 'clonus,' manifested by rhythmic repeated contraction of the hyperreflexic muscle when stretch is suddenly applied and maintained.

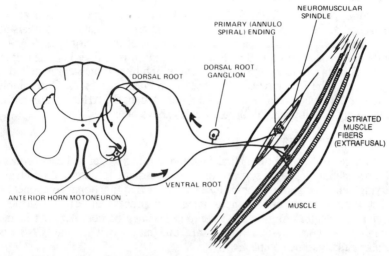

FIGURE 56. Muscle stretch reflex. This is a monosynaptic reflex, with only one central synapse.

TONE; TONUS

In neurology, these terms ordinarily refer to the resistance to passive movement about a joint due to abnormal muscular activity. Tonus may be increased or decreased because of a variety of CNS changes causing alterations in muscle activity. Spasticity or hyperreflexia is one example of hypertonus, due to UMN lesions. Lower motor neuron lesions cause flaccidity or hypotonus, with decreased muscle stretch reflexes.

Decreased reflexes with LMN lesions result from loss of effector ventral root axons, with resultant decrease in reflex muscle contraction.

GAMMA MOTOR SYSTEM

Gamma motor (efferent) system refers to small anterior horn motoneurons and their fine myelinated axons (Table 7) projecting not to somatic extrafusal muscle but to small muscle fibers within the neuromuscular spindle itself (intrafusal muscle fibers). Extrafusal muscle fibers provide the force of contraction of a muscle. Intrafusal fibers provide no contractile force, rather they act to change the level of excitability of the muscle stretch reflex.

Primary endings in the central zone of intrafusal muscle fibers respond to sudden stretch, acting as the receptor for muscle stretch reflex. Secondary endings in the spindle are concerned with constant, tonic, postural muscular stretch and contraction (Figure 57).

During normal muscular activity, gamma anterior horn cells are continuously stimulated by various inputs. Intrafusal muscle fibers therefore remain partially contracted — i.e., some of them are contracted most of the time. This means that the gamma system can become either more or less active, thus increasing or decreasing the muscle stretch reflex. In particular, overactivity of the gamma system accounts for much of the spasticity of UMN lesions, and underactivity may cause hypotonus, as with cerebellar lesions.

Through a feedback function of the gamma efferent system, volitional movement may be smoothed (Figure 58). The pyramidal tract usually excites both alpha and gamma motoneurons so that intrafusal and extrafusal muscle fibers contract equally. This is called alpha-gamma coactivation. If the movement initiated by the pyramidal tract meets an unforeseen load, muscle shortening stops or slows, while intrafusal muscle fibers continue to increase tension on their central zones, thus inducing a reflex increase of the force of contraction. This occurs at the spinal level, requires no cerebral input, and takes much less time (about 25 msec) than volitional correction for the increased load, which requires 100 msec or more.

If, in contrast, the load on the muscle is unexpectedly lightened, shortening of the muscle as a whole speeds up, decreasing tension on the neuromuscular spindle, turning off the response of the primary ending, and reflexly decreasing the strength of contraction.

GOLGI TENDON ORGAN

Neuromuscular spindles operate in parallel with extrafusal muscle fibers (Figures 56 and 58). Golgi tendon organs (GTO), on the other hand, act in series (see Figure 59). GTOs have a well-known emergency function—inhibition of strong contractions that might rupture the muscle. They are also involved in normal movement, as follows.

For postural control, tension on the GTO maintains a constant, tonic flow of inhibitory impulses onto AHC. When tension decreases, GTO

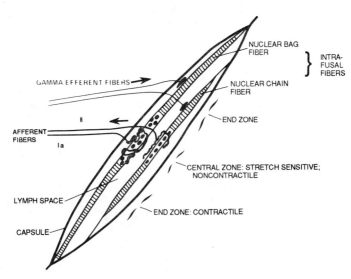

FIGURE 57. Neuromuscular spindle. Afferent Ia fibers carry action potentials induced in primary endings on nuclear bag fibers by stretch. II fibers carry impulses from secondary endings on nuclear chain fibers, responding tonically to length. The drawing is simplified; intrafusal fibers usually number 6 to 14.

inhibition decreases, and AHC become more active, returning the muscle tension toward its original level. When tension increases, GTO inhibiltion increases, decreasing AHC activity and decreasing muscle tension, again toward its original level.

Thus, unloading of muscle tension facilitates rapid movement through GTO function. At the spinal level, the golgi tendon organ and the neuromuscular spindle smooth movement by feedback mechanisms working in opposite directions.

SUPERFICIAL REFLEXES — Flexor Withdrawal Reflexes

In the normal human, stimulation of the foot often leads to reflex withdrawal, especially if the stimulus is noxious or painful. This flexor withdrawal reflex is polysynaptic, in contrast to the monosynaptic muscle stretch reflex. A clinically important example is the Babinski reflex, which consists of dorsiflexion of the big toe when the bottom of the foot is gently scratched. It is seen in adults with pyramidal tract (UMN) lesions.

Nonpainful stimulation of the foot in adults normally causes downward, plantar, flexion of the big toe. This normal plantar response is part of the walking mechanism, and is maintained by the pyramidal tract. The Babinski reflex occurs in response to gentle plantar stimulation only when the spinal cord acts autonomously, i.e., when the pyramidal tract is damaged, preventing descent of cerebral influences (Figure 60).

Babinski reflex is normal in babies. Until they walk, the pyramidal tract remains incompletely myelinated and only partially functional. Myelination

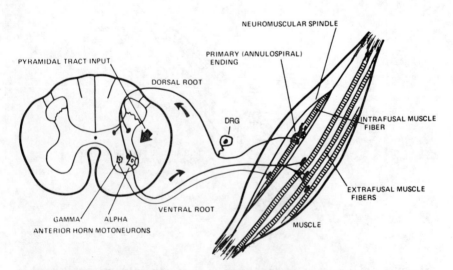

FIGURE 58. Gamma motor feedback loop. Impulses from gamma anterior horn cells, evoked by pyramidal tract or other inputs, cause contraction of intrafusal muscle fibers, partially stretching the central zone, and increasing the muscle stretch fibers.

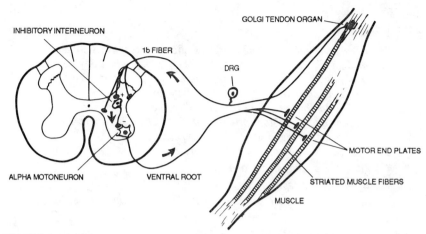

FIGURE 59. Golgi tendon organ. Contraction of the muscle stretches the tendon and attached GTO, initiating action potentials which inhibit alpha motoneurons by way of inhibitory interneurons.

perfects pyramidal tract function, and walking becomes possible. At the same time, the tract activates the interneurons which inhibit the infantile Babinski response.

UMN lesions also cause loss of three other superficial reflexes: abdominal skin reflex; cremasteric reflex; and anal reflex. For the first, gently scratching abdominal skin causes contraction of the underlying abdominal muscle. For the cremasteric reflex, scratching the scrotum or inner thigh causes elevation of the ipsilateral testis. Scratching perineal skin causes puckering of the anal sphincter — the anal reflex.

MOTOR PATTERNS

To summarize: A specific movement begins with descent of complex patterned volleys of action potentials from the cortex along the pyramidal tract and other routes, to synapse with spinal cord alpha and gamma AHC, and with excitatory and inhibitory interneurons. These impulses cause rhythmic contraction of motor units of the primary (agonist) muscle and of the synergistic muscles needed for the movement, together with simultaneous inhibition of antagonists. The same volleys adjust the reflex reactivity of alpha AHC and of the gamma system and GTO to smooth the contraction.

In human motor function, the importance of the pyramidal tract is worth additional emphasis, both in its own right and as the common pathway along which many other systems project to the lower motor neuron.

CLINICAL EXAMPLE 11

A man brought to the emergency room unconscious after an auto accident had a right scalp laceration and a skull fracture, demonstrated by x-ray. No muscle stretch reflexes could be elicited.

The next day, however, his left knee jerk and ankle jerk were much more active than the right, and he showed a left Babinski sign.

Discussion

The absence of muscle stretch reflexes after head injury is called cerebral shock, usually a temporary state, lasting only a day in this instance. Hyperactive left knee and ankle jerks (spasticity) suggest an upper motor neuron lesion, with partial loss of descending inhibitory influences, probably due to damage to the right motor and premotor cortex (areas 4 and 6). This interpretation was supported by the observed left Babinski.

This patient demonstrated the three cardinal findings of UMN lesions:

(1) Paralysis or paresis (weakness);

(2) Hyperreflexia (spasticity); and

(3) Babinski sign, often associated with changes in other superficial reflexes.

CLINICAL EXAMPLE 12

A young woman came to the physician's office because of diplopia that had begun about 6 months earlier. More recently, her arms and legs had become weak. She observed that, after resting, she could work fairly normally for a time, but gradually got weaker and weaker and soon could scarcely move. She was given a tensilon test, and proved to have myasthenia gravis.

Discussion

Diplopia or double vision may result from weakness of extraocular muscles. In myasthenia gravis, the motor end plate is damaged by an autoimmune mechanism, so that its neurotransmitter (acetylcholine = ACh), is ineffective, and muscle contraction becomes weak.

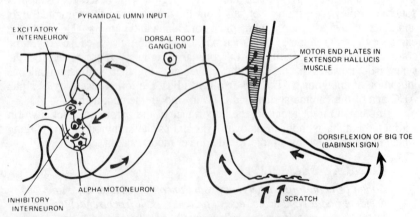

FIGURE 60. Babinski reflex. When the UMN input to inhibitory interneurons is lost, stimulation of the sole of the foot elicits a spinal reflex of flexor withdrawal type. The first evidence of this withdrawal is dorsiflexion of the big toe, the Babinski reflex.

Treatment with anticholinesterase drugs, which slow down the normal enzymatic destruction of ACh, increases the amount of neurotransmitter available, and so increases muscle strength. Tensilon (edrophonium) is a drug of this type with a very transient effect so that it can be used to test for the disease. If the patient is myasthenic, a dramatic but brief increase in strength follows the test injection of tensilon.

CLINICAL EXAMPLE 13

In the days before polio vaccine, a girl age 12 contracted polio involving her left quadriceps muscles. As the acute phase passed, extension at the left knee (quadriceps function) was very weak, and the left knee jerk was almost absent. Examined three months later, in addition to the weakness and decreased reflex, the left quadriceps was only about 10% of its original size. Discuss.

Discussion

The polio virus destroys anterior horn motoneurons. This young lady demonstrated the three major findings of lower motor neuron (LMN) lesions, in this instance involving only the quadriceps muscle:

(1) Paralysis or paresis;

(2) Flaccidity with hyporeflexia; and

(3) Muscle atrophy.

Contrast these findings with the UMN findings of Example 11.

CLINICAL EXAMPLE 14

A young man severely hyperflexed his neck in a diving accident. Brought to the emergency room, his arms and legs were paralyzed and flaccid. Muscle stretch reflexes gradually increased, and eventually became hyperactive (spastic). Two months later he was still able to move only his right toes and his left arm.

Discussion

Neck hyperflexion damaged his cervical spinal cord. Immediate flaccidity resulted from spinal shock (see Clinical Example 11), with later development of spasticity. Inability to move three extremities (triplegia) was due to the upper motor neuron lesion. Paralysis of one extremity is called monoplegia, of both legs paraplegia, of half the body hemiplegia, and of all four extremities, quadriplegia. Bilateral Babinski reflexes would also be expected.

STUDY QUESTIONS

1. Diagram the course of the pyramidal tract, from cortex to spinal cord, with labels.
2. What are the giant pyramidal cells of Betz?
3. Discuss the presence of a Babinski reflex in a baby who is not yet able to walk.
4. Account for the spasticity (hyperreflexia) of UMN lesions.
5. Account for the flaccidity of LMN lesions.
6. What is a neuromuscular spindle? How does it function?
7. What is the gamma motor system? How does it operate to smooth volitional movement?
8. Define: Reflex, UMN, LMN, internal capsule.
9. Describe how volitional movement occurs, starting with the cortical origin of the pyramidal tract. Pick an uncomplicated movement to discuss.
10. What is a motor unit?
11. What is meant by volitional (voluntary) movement? Discuss this important question in anatomical and in functional terms.
12. What are the three major signs of UMN lesions?
13. What are the three major signs of LMN lesion?

7 Somatic Sensory Systems

Somatic sensation has been divided into a number of modalities: touch, pain of two types, position sense, kinesthetic sense, warmth, cold, vibration sense, pressure. Around 1900, investigators believed that each modality was mediated by a specific anatomical type of sensory receptor ending. For a time in the 1940s, this was denied, but recent work suggests that the earlier ideas of function and anatomical specificity are mostly correct.

GENERAL PATTERNS

From peripheral receptor to sensory cortex, the basic sensory pathway consists of three neurons (Figure 61).

Impulses travel centripetally from the peripheral receptor toward the cell body of the first-order neuron in the dorsal root ganglion of the spinal nerve. Its axon extends centrally to synapse with second-order neurons in the posterior horn of the spinal cord, or in homologous nuclei of the brain stem. Axons of the second-order neurons cross the midline, and ascend on the opposite side as the spinothalamic tract or medial lemniscus, to the next synapse in the thalamus. Thalamic neurons, usually third-order, lie in the ventrobasal complex (VB) of the thalamus, and project via the posterior limb of the internal capsule to the sensory cortex of the postcentral gyrus (Brodmann's areas 3-1-2; see Figures 62 and 63).

This pattern emphasizes several important points:

1. The system is crossed. Sensory information from one half of the body projects to the opposite thalamus and cortex (note parallel with pyramidal tract).

2. First-order neurons are in dorsal root ganglia.

3. Cell bodies of second-order neurons are in the posterior horn of the spinal cord or in homologous nuclei, such as nucleus gracilis from leg or cuneatus from arm (dorsal column nuclei) of the medulla.

4. Third-order neurons in the thalamus relay impulses to the cortex.

PUNCTATE INNERVATION — THE HOMUNCULUS

Each point on the skin projects sensory information via a single fiber pathway to a single point on the sensory cortex. The pattern produced by this punctate (point-to-point) representation forms a distorted cortical homunculus (Latin = doll) — see Figure 63.

Areas of cortical projections are directly proportional to the numbers of neurons innervating the specific body region. Correlated with highly concentrated innervation of thumb and tongue are the large cortical representations of these structures (Figure 63).

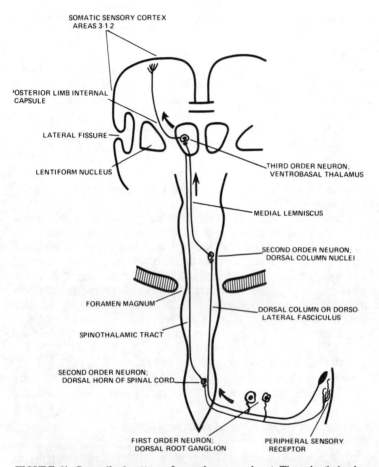

SOMATIC SENSORY CORTEX
AREAS 3·1·2

POSTERIOR LIMB INTERNAL
CAPSULE

LATERAL FISSURE

LENTIFORM NUCLEUS

THIRD ORDER NEURON;
VENTROBASAL THALAMUS

MEDIAL LEMNISCUS

SECOND ORDER NEURON;
DORSAL COLUMN NUCLEI

FORAMEN MAGNUM

DORSAL COLUMN OR DORSO·
LATERAL FASCICULUS

SPINOTHALAMIC TRACT

SECOND ORDER NEURON;
DORSAL HORN OF SPINAL CORD

FIRST ORDER NEURON;
DORSAL ROOT GANGLION

PERIPHERAL SENSORY
RECEPTOR

FIGURE 61. Generalized pattern of somatic sensory input. The spinothalamic route is usual for pain and temperature sensibility (see also Figure 70). Fibers relaying in dorsal column nuclei mediate proprioceptive sensations (see Figure 71). Touch travels by both routes.

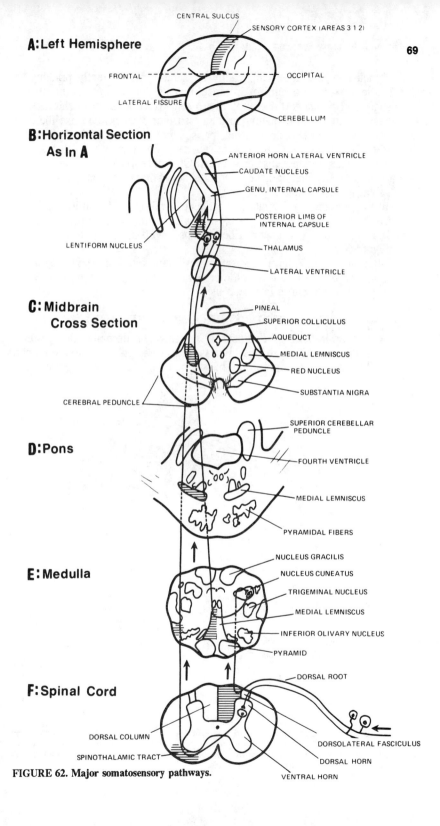

FIGURE 62. Major somatosensory pathways.

A: Left Hemisphere

CENTRAL SULCUS
SENSORY CORTEX (AREAS 3 1 2)
FRONTAL
OCCIPITAL
LATERAL FISSURE
CEREBELLUM

69

B: Horizontal Section As In A

ANTERIOR HORN LATERAL VENTRICLE
CAUDATE NUCLEUS
GENU, INTERNAL CAPSULE
POSTERIOR LIMB OF INTERNAL CAPSULE
LENTIFORM NUCLEUS
THALAMUS
LATERAL VENTRICLE

C: Midbrain Cross Section

PINEAL
SUPERIOR COLLICULUS
AQUEDUCT
MEDIAL LEMNISCUS
RED NUCLEUS
SUBSTANTIA NIGRA
CEREBRAL PEDUNCLE

D: Pons

SUPERIOR CEREBELLAR PEDUNCLE
FOURTH VENTRICLE
MEDIAL LEMNISCUS
PYRAMIDAL FIBERS

E: Medulla

NUCLEUS GRACILIS
NUCLEUS CUNEATUS
TRIGEMINAL NUCLEUS
MEDIAL LEMNISCUS
INFERIOR OLIVARY NUCLEUS
PYRAMID

F: Spinal Cord

DORSAL ROOT
DORSAL COLUMN
DORSOLATERAL FASCICULUS
SPINOTHALAMIC TRACT
DORSAL HORN
VENTRAL HORN

Punctate organization can readily be demonstrated. Gently pricking the skin of the wrist with a pin, for instance, reveals that at some points the pin feels sharp and at others it does not. Sharp-sensitive points lie much closer together on fingertips, lips, or tongue than on trunk or neck, because there are more sensory nerve fibers and endings per square millimeter in the former than the latter. Two-point discrimination is tested by simultaneous touch with two fine, blunt points variable distances apart. On fingertips and tongue, points 1 mm apart are easily distinguished. On the back, points 3-5 cm apart may still be felt as a single stimulus.

In the projection schemata of Figures 61 and 62, an incoming (afferent) dorsal root fiber is depicted as synapsing with a single neuron in the spinal cord. In actual fact, each sensory fiber synapses with up to 300 neurons in the cord (Figure 64).

Multiple sensory terminals serve important inter- and intrasegmental functions, just as do those of the motor pyramidal tract, through synapses on excitatory and on inhibitory interneurons.

LATERAL INHIBITION (SURROUND INHIBITION)

A function important in all sensory systems, and in many other systems, is lateral inhibition. Through this process, sensory impulses maintain emphasis and discreteness by inhibition of surrounding neuronal impulse transmission.

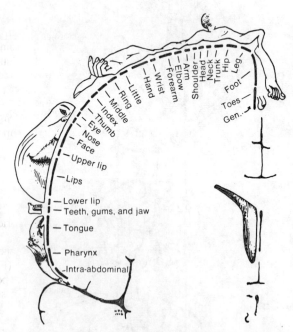

FIGURE 63. Diagram showing the relative size of the parts of the postcentral cortex from which sensations localized to different parts of the body can be elicited on electrical stimulation in man. (Reproduced, with permission, from Penfield and Rasmussen: *The Cerebral Cortex of Man*, MacMillan, New York, 1950)

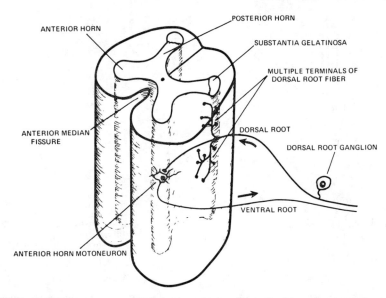

FIGURE 64. Multiple axon terminals of a dorsal root afferent fiber in gray matter of spinal cord. Drawing is simplified — the total number of endings may reach several hundred.

In Figure 65, a sensory impulse arriving from the right synaptically activates the direct sensory relay neuron (C) to initiate a centripetal ascending action potential, indicated by the arrow going up to the left. The same impulse activates adjacent inhibitory interneurons to decrease the activity of surrounding sensory relay neurons (A), (B), (D), and (E), so that no action potentials are relayed (Os on the left). Thus the relayed impulse (C) stands out against a surround of neuronal inactivity.

Lateral or surround inhibition occurs at all levels of all mammalian sensory systems. Here again we see an example of the great importance of inhibition in CNS function.

SENSORY RECEPTOR ENDINGS

Specialized nerve terminals in skin, subcutaneous tissue, periosteum, joint capsules, and elsewhere respond to various types of sensory stimulation. These endings may be classified into three broad anatomical categories, though intermediate forms are common (Table 9).

Free nerve endings appear under the electron microscope as fine unmyelinated nerve fibers among the cells of the innervated tissue (Figure 66). A thin layer of Schwann cell cytoplasm surrounds the fibers except perhaps for their very tips. Fine endings occur in almost every body tissue, subserving pain and other modalities.

TABLE 9. Anatomical categories of sensory endings

1. Free nerve endings.
2. Hederiform endings, with bulbous terminations.
3. Encapsulated endings.

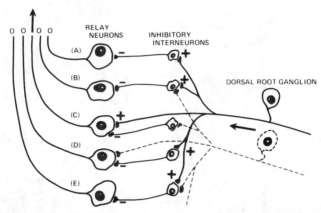

FIGURE 65. Lateral inhibition, sharpening a sensory impulse entering the spinal cord from the right. + indicates excitatory synapses; — indicates inhibitory synapses; ---- shows the parallel pathways of an adjacent sensory neuron. 0 means absence of action potential in the fibers indicated.

Hederiform (ivy-shaped) endings also exist in many locations, as unencapsulated terminal swellings on fine nerve fibers. They are usually at least partially surrounded by Schwann cell cytoplasm, and may make intimate contact with epithelial cells. The type example is Merkel's disc in the epidermis (Figure 66).

The type example of encapsulated endings is the pacinian corpuscle, whose terminal sensory fiber lies inside a bulb of onion-skin layers of connective tissue (Figures 66 and 67). Similar but smaller Golgi-Mazzoni endings in joint capsules respond to movement and tension.

Meissner's corpuscles, also encapsulated (Figure 66) lie in dermal papillae in hands and feet to mediate touch. Their capsule incorporates cells apparently of Schwann derivation, separating fine nerve terminals. Intermediate forms (Figure 66) appear in various regions, and similar genital corpuscles are found in the mucous membrane of the glans. Other variants such as the endings of Krause appear to mediate warmth or cold sensations.

In hairy regions of the skin, complex palisades of nerve endings surround hair follicles and mediate the delicate sensibility of hair movement.

Thus, considerable evidence suggests that specific sensations may be mediated by specific endings, but with many important exceptions. The most often cited exception is the cornea of the eye where only free nerve endings exist; yet touch, pain, warmth, and cold sensations are appreciated. In addition, overstimulation of almost any ending, particularly if noxious, may induce painful sensations.

GENERATOR POTENTIALS

Every sensory receptor transduces physical stimuli into action potentials. Neurophysiological investigations have shown that the adequate stimulus (touch, pressure, warmth, vibration, etc.) provokes the development of an electrical potential across the membrane of the sensory terminal, probably through a change in ionic permeabilities. These generator potentials are graded, i.e., they are not all-or-none events: the more intense the stimulus, the larger the resultant generator potential.

Generator potentials have been studied most intensively in pacinian corpuscles because of their large size (up to several millimeters), their well-defined capsule, and the ease with which mechanical stimuli can be quantitated. Here has been most clearly demonstrated the direct relation between strength of stimulus and the potential generated. If the generator potential from the mechanically deformed central fiber exceeds threshold at the first node of Ranvier, which usually lies within the capsule, then a propagated action potential is initiated (Figure 67).

Generator potentials similar to Figure 67 occur at most sensory endings, initiating propagated potentials if threshold is exceeded. Generator potentials from different endings differ in duration and rate of adaptation. A long-continued stimulus may result in a generator potential of long duration, tonic or slowly-

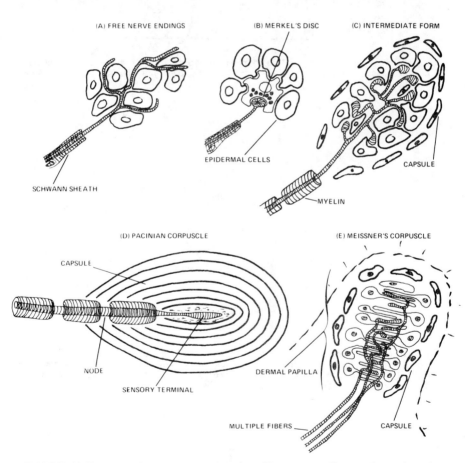

FIGURE 66. Examples of sensory receptor endings. Free nerve endings mediate pain and other sensations, pacinian corpuscles mediate pressure and vibration, Meissner's and Merkel's endings mediate touch. There are many intermediate forms.

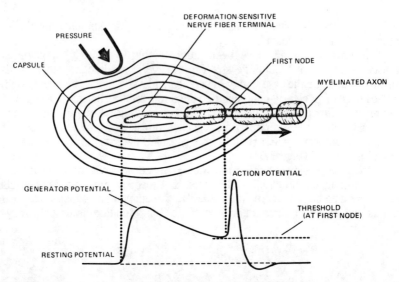

FIGURE 67. Generator potential in response to deformation of a pacinian corpuscle. Threshold was exceeded at the first node, initiating an action potential which propagates to the right.

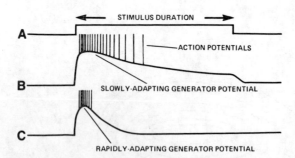

FIGURE 68. Tonic and phasic sensory responses. (A) A long-continued stimulus. (B) Tonic response; long series of action potentials because of the slow decrement of the generator potential. (C) Phasic response; short sequence of action potentials, because of rapid adaptation of generator potential, which quickly falls below threshold.

adapting, or one which decrements rapidly, phasic or rapidly-adapting (see Figure 68).

Clothing which has been in place for a couple of minutes is no longer felt. The phasic touch receptors stimulated on donning the clothing cease to respond after brief adaptation. In contrast, some stimuli, such as the pain of toothache or postural sense from joints act on tonic receptors and remain perceptible after minutes or hours of unchanging stimulation.

SENSORY CODING

Sensory inputs can be defined, coded, in terms of three parameters: location, intensity, and modality. Coding for location (review Figures 63 and 69) can be considered segmentally. Dorsal root fibers entering each spinal segment transmit impulses from a specific region of skin, a dermatome; from specific muscles, a myotome; and from specific bony and joint regions, a sclerotome. In neck and trunk, these three regions correspond. In limbs and head, however, they do not correspond because of distortions of our primeval tube-like body organization during development. The pattern of dermatomes is sketched in Figure 69.

CLINICAL EXAMPLE 15

A 45-year-old woman came to the hospital with fever, nausea, pain in the right shoulder and root of neck, and a history of indigestion from fatty foods. Acute cholecystitis (inflammation of the gall bladder) was diagnosed, with irradiation of the underside of her right diaphragm. The neck and shoulder pain was referred pain.

Discussion

Innervation of the diaphragm by the phrenic nerve arises from C3 to C5. By Figure 69, these dermatomes cover the lower neck and shoulder. Pain impulses from the irritated diaphragm enter the cord at C3 to C5 and synapse with sensory neurons also receiving inputs from neck and shoulder. This overlap or convergence is interpreted centrally as pain coming from the shoulder. Synaptic convergence probably accounts for most if not all referred sensation.

CODING FOR INTENSITY OF STIMULATION

The more intense a sensory stimulus, the higher the frequency of afferent potentials. Recruitment of increased numbers of action potentials for intensity coding occurs through two mechanisms: increased frequency of potentials from a single ending, and through increased numbers of activated endings. Note the similarity of this process to the control of strength of muscle contraction discussed earlier.

SENSORY MODALITY

In a clinical setting, or in the laboratory, confusion in defining sensory modalities can be avoided by specifying the method of stimulation. To avoid the philosophic problem of defining pain for example, the sentence 'pin-prick sensation was decreased in the right hand' informs unambiguously.

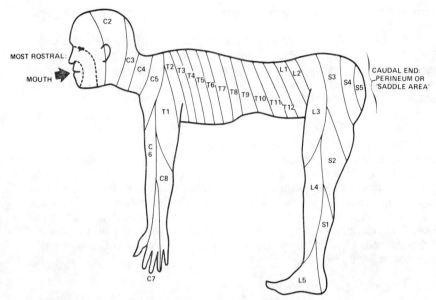

FIGURE 69. Pattern of dermatomes. Note that the saddle area is most caudal and the mouth most rostral of the dermatomes. Face is supplied by the trigeminal (fifth cranial) nerve. Other useful relations to remember: shoulder is C5; hand is C6-C7-C8; nipple is T4; umbilicus is T10; foot is L4-L5-S1; saddle area is S3-S4-S5.

CLINICAL EXAMPLE 16

A middle-aged man was diagnosed on clinical and laboratory grounds as having a tumor of the cauda equina with damage to nerve roots S3, 4, 5. What signs and symptoms would you expect?

Discussion

From Figure 69, S3, 4, 5 innervate the saddle area, including the perineum, where sensory and motor loss would disturb normal function of bladder and anal sphincters. Therefore, the patient's earliest difficulties would likely be urinary and/or fecal incontinence or retention, resulting from motor loss with inability to contract and relax the sphincters, and from sensory loss with inability to detect fullness of bladder and rectum. Review Figures 6 and 69.

PAIN - TEMPERATURE PATHWAYS

Pain and temperature impulses ascend the same pathway in the spinal cord. Beginning with appropriate stimulation of receptor endings, action potentials pass centripetally to first-order neurons in dorsal root ganglia then, via dorsal roots, into the cord. These are mostly fine, often unmyelinated nerve fibers (types III and IV, Table 5) which enter the cord in the lateral portion of the dorsal root (Figure 70). They immediately ascend a couple of segments in the dorsolateral fasciculus (Lissauer), then turn into the posterior horn to synapse with second-order sensory neurons, in or deep to the substantia gelatinosa (in Rexed's laminae I and II and in deeper layers IV and V — see Figure 72). Axons of these second-order sensory neurons cross the midline as the anterior white commissure just ventral to the central canal of the cord, then turn rostrally, ascending to the brain stem as the spinothalamic tract in the anterolateral column of the cord (Figures 61, 62, and 70). Within the brain stem, the fibers mediating the primitive, diffuse, unlocalized, 'global' kind of pain apparently relay via neurons in the reticular formation of medulla and pons and periaqueductal gray matter of the midbrain to the intralaminar nuclei of the thalamus. This is the emotionally distressing kind of pain experienced on barking one's shin, or breaking a bone. Its cortical projection may be to the orbital gyri of the frontal lobe.

The other kind of pain, better called pin-prick sensibility, is very accurately localized via a direct pathway from cord through brain stem to the VPL (ventro-postero-lateral part of the ventrobasal thalamus), thence to sensory cortex, areas 3-1-2, Figures 61, 62, and 70.

Clinical and experimental observations suggest that perception of pain mostly occurs at thalamic rather than cortical levels, though its localization is cortical (compare Clinical Example 17). Electrical stimulation of sensory cortex seldom provokes subjective pain.

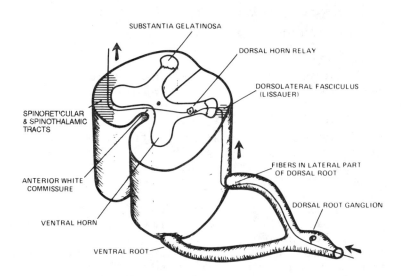

SUBSTANTIA GELATINOSA

DORSAL HORN RELAY

DORSOLATERAL FASCICULUS (LISSAUER)

SPINORET'CULAR & SPINOTHALAMIC TRACTS

FIBERS IN LATERAL PART OF DORSAL ROOT

ANTERIOR WHITE COMMISSURE

DORSAL ROOT GANGLION

VENTRAL HORN

VENTRAL ROOT

FIGURE 70. Pain-temperature pathway from the periphery into the ascending spinothalamic-spinoreticular tracts in the anterolateral quadrant of the spinal cord. (Compare Figure 62.)

CLINICAL EXAMPLE 17

An elderly gentleman had a stroke, fell, and found himself unable to move his left arm. Gradually, arm movement improved, and on examination a week later, the most prominent finding was excruciating pain in the left shoulder and upper arm. The slightest touch caused grimacing and groans. Sensation in the same region was decreased. This is called a thalamic syndrome.

Discussion

The gentleman undoubtedly suffered a CVA (cerebrovascular accident) with infarction in his right posterior thalamus. Motor connections in the area were somewhat damaged, causing weakness, but damage to pain pathways was more serious. The severely distressing nature of the discomfort suggests that the primitive pain system was mainly damaged, probably with disinhibition and resultant overreaction.

WITHDRAWAL REFLEXES; Polysynaptic Spinal Reflexes

As discussed in the previous chapter, noxious stimulation of an extremity commonly causes reflex withdrawal. In contrast to the monosynaptic muscle stretch reflex, the withdrawal reflexes are polysynaptic, including two or more central synapses. Because of this multiplicity of synaptic interactions, the reflexes are usually more labile than muscle stretch reflexes. They often involve multiple segments.

The Babinski reflex (Figure 60) is an example of a withdrawal reflex of pathologic significance.

CROSSED EXTENSOR REFLEX

Simultaneously with withdrawal from a noxious stimulus, the opposite extremity often extends, aiding in the removal of the injured extremity from its noxious environment, This crossed-extensor reflex is mediated by interneuronal connections from the side of stimulation to extensor AHC on the other side. A similar crossed reflex makes up part of the sequence of normal walking.

PROPRIOCEPTIVE PATHWAY

Proprioception (Latin = self-sensation) is the name applied to joint position sense, kinesthetic sense, vibration sense, and some aspects of topognosis, (identification of location of the body). Impulses originate peripherally in pacinian corpuscles and other endings in joints, ligaments, dermis, and periosteum.

Proprioceptive axons, with cell bodies in dorsal root ganglia, enter the cord in the medial part of the dorsal root and ascend in the adjacent posterior and dorsolateral columns of the cord: fasciculus gracilis from the leg; fasciculus cuneatus from the arm. They synapse on second-order neurons in dorsal column nuclei (nuclei gracilis and cuneatus) in the medulla (Figures 61, 62, and 71).

These are the longest neurons in humans. With afferent limbs (dendrites) beginning at the foot, perikarya in lumbosacral dorsal root ganglia, and axons ascending to the medulla, they may total 150 cm or longer.

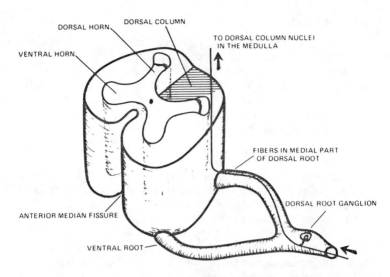

FIGURE 71. Proprioceptive pathway from periphery via posterior column (fasciculi gracilis and cuneatus). As in Figure 70, only ascending pathways are shown; the multiple intra- and intersegmental and descending branches are omitted for simplicity. (Compare Figure 62.)

MEDIAL LEMNISCUS

Nuclei gracilis and cuneatus are homologous with the dorsal horns of the spinal cord (Figure 61). Second-order axons from these nuclei sweep across the midline of the medulla in bundles often called internal arcuate fibers, to form the medial lemniscus on the opposite side (Figure 62). This decussation is homologous with the anterior white commissure of the pain-temperature system in the cord (Figure 70).

In the dorsal column nuclei occurs an important sensorimotor interaction. Collaterals from pyramidal tract fibers, arising from the sensory cortex (Figure 50) synapse with neurons in the dorsal column nuclei to modify proprioceptive information from joints and other tissues. Here a major motor system, the pyramidal tract, influences one of the major sensory inputs concerned with motor control.

Proprioceptive medial lemniscus fibers ascend further to the ventral posterolateral (VPL) nucleus of the thalamus, there to relay via third-order thalamic neurons to sensory cortex, areas 3-1-2 of the postcentral gyrus. These thalamocortical inputs run in the posterior limb of the internal capsule (see Figure 62). Different sensory modalities project to different strips of the sensory cortex, as follows:

Area 3a— Neuromuscular spindles and Golgi tendon organs.

Area 3b — Slowly adapting cutaneous receptors.

Area 1 — Rapidly-adapting cutaneous receptors, such as pacinian corpuscles.

Area 2 — Joint receptors and other deep receptors.

TOUCH PATHWAYS

Meissner's corpuscles in dermal papillae, Merkel's discs in the epidermis, and other endings mediate sensations of touch (Figure 66). Some touch fibers follow a crossed route similar to the pain-temperature pathway while others travel up the cord by the proprioceptive route, finally crossing to the other side in the medulla (Figures 61 and 62). As a result of this double routing, partial cord lesions frequently do not cause clinical loss of touch, even when other sensory modalities are disturbed.

CLINICAL EXAMPLE 18

A 24-year-old man brought to the emergency room had a stab wound in the middle of his back, at vertebral level T10. His legs were flaccid and paralyzed, with diminished sensation.

A few days later, examination showed spastic paralysis of the left leg; left Babinski reflex; loss of position sense in left toes; ankle and knee position sense normal; loss of pin-prick sensibility in right foot, grading to normal at mid-thigh; a feeling of a 'tight band' around his lower abdomen.

Where is the lesion? Account for the findings.

Discussion

Spinal cord injury is suggested by the history. Immediate flaccid paralysis followed by left spastic paralysis suggests spinal shock due to a left upper motor neuron lesion. The Babinski sign confirms this. Loss of position sense in the left toes suggests a partial left posterior column lesion. Loss of pin-prick sense on the right suggests a left spinothalamic tract lesion. No findings were more rostral than the lower abdomen, so that the lesion must have been at that level or higher. The feeling of a 'tight band' supports this. This is the syndrome of cord hemisection, or a Brown-Sequard syndrome, at cord level L1 or T12, corresponding to vertebral level T10.

The three cardinal signs of the Brown-Sequard syndrome, as seen in this patient are:

(1) Paralysis on the same side as the lesion.

(2) Proprioceptive loss, also ipsilateral; and

(3) Pain and temperature loss on the opposite side.

Touch is often not affected, and the three changes listed occur caudal to the level of the lesion. Occasionally, there will also be signs or symptoms at the level of the lesion, as with this patient.

LAMINATION OF LONG TRACTS

Each of the long tracts so far discussed is organized in layers or laminae corresponding to dermatomes (Figure 72). The laminar organization results from the way the tracts are built up, namely by accretion of fibers to the near side of the tract. This lamination may be of medical significance, as in Clinical Example 19.

LAMINATION OF SPINAL CORD GRAY MATTER

Gray matter of the spinal cord can be subdivided into functional and anatomical laminae.The system most widely used was introduced by Rexed (Figure 72).

CLINICAL EXAMPLE 19

Six months before admission, a 38-year-old man developed constipation and partial loss of libido, followed in a couple of weeks by tingling of the left foot, weakness of the right foot, increasing constipation, and occasional urinary incontinence. After treating himself with cathartics for a time, he saw a urologist because of the incontinence, and was referred for neurological study. Unfortunately, in the 10 days between referral and arrival at the hospital, motor function in his legs had grossly deteriorated. Findings on admission: urinary incontinence, loss of nearly all sensation in the saddle area and both legs, spastic paraplegia, bilateral Babinski reflexes. Account for the sequence of clinical signs.

Discussion

As in this instance, the first sign of spinal cord tumor may be change in urinary or bowel function, though obviously these are more often due to non-neurological conditions. Sphincters are involved early

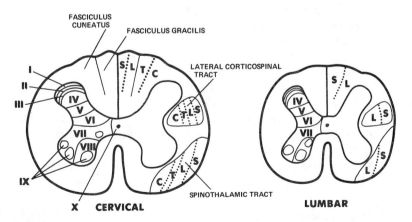

FIGURE 72. Cervical and lumbar spinal cord sections. Right side—lamination of posterior column, pyramidal tract, and spinothalamic tract. S = sacral; L = lumbar; T = thoracic; C = cervical cord. Left side of sections—lamination of gray matter according to Rexed. Lamina II is the substantia gelatinosa and lamina IX consists of islands of motoneurons.

because lamination of sensory and motor pathways for the saddle area lie superficially in the cord (see Figure 72), and are likely to be damaged early by external pressure. With this patient, as the tumor enlarged, it damaged deeper layers, and the legs lost motor and sensory function.

The findings given suggest a low thoracic (T11-T12) tumor. Myelography or computerized axial tomography (CAT scan) would localize it more accurately in preparation for surgical removal.

CLINICAL EXAMPLE 20

A 25-year-old man observed that his cigarette burned his finger without causing pain. In fact, he was unaware that he had been burned until he smelled scorching skin! On examination there was grossly diminished pain sense (pin-prick and periosteal) in the middle three fingers of both hands. No other abnormalities were found. Touch, motor function, and joint sense were normal in both hands. Account for this sensory dissociation.

Discussion

Spinal cord level C7 corresponds to the middle fingers. Examination of Figures 62 and 70 suggests that dissociated loss of pain without loss of other sensory modalities could result from damage to crossing pain fibers of the anterior white commissure. Such a lesion may result from syringomyelia, a pathologic process in which the central canal of the cord becomes patent and expands, destroying the crossing fibers.

STUDY QUESTIONS

1. Draw a labeled cross-section of the spinal cord at the upper thoracic level, showing major long tracts.
2. Diagram and label the complete pathways for:
   —Pain-temperature sensibility
   —proprioception
   —touch.
3. What is the Brown-Sequard syndrome? Cite the three major findings supporting this diagnosis.
4. What is meant by lateral or surround inhibition? Give two examples.
5. In a sensory receptor, what is a generator potential? How does it develop?
6. Describe the topographic relationship between sensation from the skin (dermatomes) and the central nervous system at various levels.
7. What is a sensory modality? Give examples.
8. How is the intensity of a sensory stimulus coded in the nervous system?
9. Describe the two pathways for pain, and their perceptual differences.

8 Brain Stem and Cranial Nerves

Those portions of the CNS which continue the segmentation of the spinal cord rostrally from the spinal cord in the embryo, namely medulla, pons, and midbrain, make up the brain stem. Cerebellum and diencephalon are occasionally included in this somewhat vague term. Cerebellum, diencephalon, and telencephalon are unsegmented structures, the cerebellum being a large dorsal outgrowth of the metencephalon, and the diencephalon and telencephalon (cerebral hemispheres) deriving from the single prosencephalic vesicle of the early embryo.

Cranial nerves III through XII are embryologically homologous with spinal nerves. The olfactory nerve (cranial nerve I) is not, developing as an early part of the primitive telencephalon. The optic nerve (cranial nerve II) is not, developing as an outpouching from the diencephalon.

After reviewing the general morphology of the brain stem (Figures 4, 96, and 97) names and functions of the twelve cranial nerves should be committed to memory (Table 10).

Cranial nerve nuclei derived originally from cell columns homologous with the columns of the spinal cord. They have been assigned embryologically determined generic names which will occasionally be used, and therefore should be familiar. Table 11 summarizes these terms, and the functions related to their cell columns.

Somatic motor means neurons controlling voluntary muscles derived from somites.

Branchial motor means neurons controlling voluntary muscles derived from embryonic gill arches.

Somatic sensory means sensation from skin, mucous membranes, joints, and teeth.

Special sensory refers to equilibrium and hearing. In a broad sense, vision and olfaction are also special senses, but they do not develop from segmental columnar anlagen.

Visceral efferent means parasympathetics to eyes, to glands, and to thoracic and abdominal viscera.

Visceral afferent refers to the sense of taste and the reflex afferents from carotid body, aortic body, and from thoracic and abdominal viscera.

OLFACTORY NERVE

Numerous fascicles containing a total of about 10,000,000 unmyelinated axons with cell bodies in the upper nasal mucosa extend through the cribriform plate of the ethmoid bone as the olfactory bulb, up to 25,000 olfactory axons per mitral cell (Figures 3 and 80). Mitral cells relay backward along the

TABLE 10. The cranial nerves; locations of nuclei and functions

	Nerve	Location of nuclei	Function
I	Olfactory	Frontal lobes	Olfactory and olfactory reflexes
II	Optic	Thalamus	Vision and visual reflexes
III	Oculomotor	Midbrain	Movement of eye, constriction of pupil, accommodation of lens
IV	Trochlear	Midbrain	Movement of eye (superior oblique)
V	Trigeminal	Midbrain	Proprioception for chewing (mesencephalic nucleus)
		Pons	Sensation from face, motor for chewing, motor to tensor tympani muscle
		Medulla	Sensation from face
VI	Abducens	Pons	Lateral movement of eye (lateral rectus)
VII	Facial	Pons	Motor for facial expression, motor to stapedius muscle
		Medulla	Taste from anterior tongue (nucleus of solitary tract), salivation and lacrimation (salivatory nucleus)
VIII	Vestibulo-cochlear	Pons and Medulla	Equilibrium and hearing
IX	Glosso-pharyngeal	Medulla	Motor for swallowing (nucleus ambiguus), parotid gland salivation (salivatory nucleus), taste from posterior tongue (nucleus of solitary tract), visceral afferents from carotid and aortic bodies (nucleus of solitary tract)
X	Vagus	Medulla	Somatic sensation from pharynx and larynx (spinal nucleus of the trigeminal), motor for swallowing (nucleus ambiguus), motor to larynx for phonation (nucleus ambiguus), parasympathetic to thoracic and abdominal viscera (dorsal motor nucleus of the vagus), taste from epiglottis (nucleus of the solitary tract)
XI	Accessory	Medulla	Motor to sternomastoid and upper trapezius muscles
XII	Hypoglossal	Medulla	Motor to the tongue

olfactory tract (about 10,000 fibers) to the opposite olfactory bulb via anterior commissure, to the parolfactory area and subcallosal gyrus via medial olfactory stria, and to the amygdala and uncus of the temporal lobe via the lateral olfactory stria.

Olfactory sensibility is carried solely by the ipsilateral lateral olfactory stria. Lesions anywhere along this path from nasal mucosa to uncus can cause unilateral anosmia (loss of the sense of smell). The thin orbital and ethmoid bones are particularly likely to fracture wilth rear-enders, especially if the person has no restraining seat-belt, with resultant permanent anosmia and often more serious complications.

OPTIC NERVE (II)

Vision is discussed in Chapter 9.

TABLE 11. Embryonic designations of cranial nerves

Derived from basal (ventral) plates of the neural tube:
Somatic motor: III, IV, VI, XII
Branchial motor: V (chewing and tensor tympani)
VII (facial expression and stapedius)
IX, X, part of XI

Derived from alar plates of neural tube:
Somatic sensory: V and X
Special sensory: VIII

Derived from intermediate columns:
Visceral efferent: III (parasympathetic)
VII (salivatory)
IX (salivatory)
X (to viscera)
Visceral afferent: VII, IX, X (taste)
IX, X (for visceral reflexes)

OCULOMOTOR, TROCHLEAR, AND ABDUCENS NERVES (III, IV, VI)

Supranuclear control of these three nerves, all concerned with eye movements, is discussed together with light and accommodation reflexes (see Chapter 9).

Oculomotor (III) nuclei of right and left sides lie close together in the ventral periaqueductal gray matter deep to the superior colliculus (Figures 73, 79, 92, and 93). The nerve's 20,000 fibers pass ventrally through RAS (Reticular Activating System — see Chapter 13) and red nucleus to exit from the interpeduncular fossa between the cerebral peduncles, whence they pass forward through the cavernous sinus (Figure 23) into the orbit.

There they innervate pupil, ciliary body, and five of the seven extraocular muscles: medial rectus, superior rectus, inferior rectus, inferior oblique, and levator palpebrae superioris (Figure 94).

The trochlear (IV) nucleus lies ventral in the periaqueductal gray somewhat caudal to the oculomotor (Figures 73, 78, 95, and 96). It consists of about 3000 fibers which loop around the periaqueductal gray to exit dorsally on the side *opposite* the nucleus, just caudal to the inferior colliculus. It supplies a single muscle, the superior oblique, on the side opposite the nucleus.

Facial colliculi, two prominences on the floor of the fourth ventricle near the midline, mark the VI abducens nucleus (Figures 73, 77, and 95). It supplies only the lateral rectus muscle. Fibers of the facial nerve loop around the VI nucleus to account for the name facial colliculus (Figures 77 and 97).

Under the pull of extraocular muscles, the eyeball rotates in its socket like a ballbearing (Figure 94).

Conjugate movements of the eyes require the contraction in varying degrees of all seven muscles of each eye. Diplopia (double vision) is the prime symptom resulting from dysfunction of any of these muscles or nerves. To determine which muscle is weak and causing the diplopia, we note that the double images will separate most widely when the eyes rotate in the direction of pull of the weak muscle.

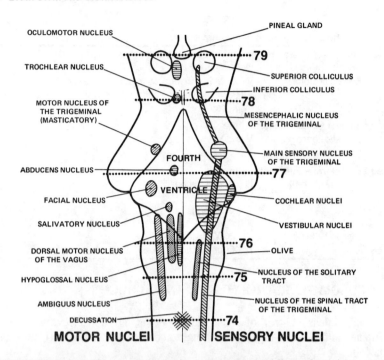

FIGURE 73. Dorsal phantom of the brain stem to show locations of cranial nerve nuclei. This figure should be correlated with Figures 4, 74-79, 95 and 96, as well as with Tables 10 and 11. Levels of sections for Figures 74-79 are indicated.

TRIGEMINAL NERVE (V)

This nerve (Latin = triplet) has 140,000 sensory fibers in three major divisions: ophthalmic (V-1), maxillary (V-2), and mandibular (V-3), supplying sensory innervation to the face (Figures 81 and 96). It is also the sensory nerve for deep structures of the head, including accessory nasal sinuses, periosteum of the skull, and intracranial dura and arteries.

Fibers of the three divisions enter the trigeminal ganglion, homologous with spinal root ganglia, at the mid-pons about 2 cm from the midline (Figures 4 and 96). Some fibers synapse in the main sensory nucleus immediately. The descending (spinal) tract of the trigeminal runs on the lateral surface of the medulla bearing sensory inputs from the face, to terminate in the spinal nucleus (Figures 73-76). Second-order axons cross the midline and ascend as ventral and dorsal trigeminal lemnisci parallel to the medial meniscus to synapse in the ventral posteromedial (VPM) thalamus (Figures 129 and 134). Third-order fibers continue via posterior limb of the internal capsule (Figures 61 and 62) to the lower end of the sensory cortex of the postcentral gyrus, areas 3-1-2.

Muscles of mastication and the tensor tympani are innervated by a small motor root of 8000 fibers, which arises from the motor nucleus just deep to the nerve's attachment. This nucleus works intimately with the mesencephalic nucleus (Figure 73), which receives proprioceptive inputs from teeth and jaws for the automatic process of chewing.

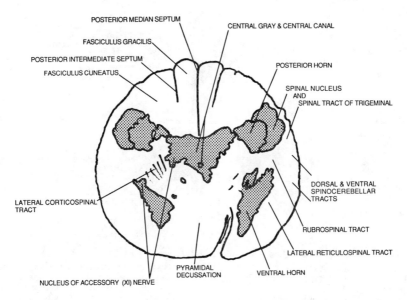

FIGURE 74. Brain stem section at the level of the pyramidal decussation; see Figure 73.

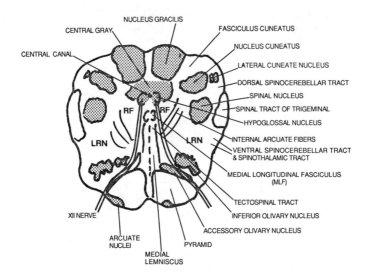

FIGURE 75. Brain stem section at the lower medulla; see Figure 73. LRN = lateral reticular nucleus; RF = reticular formation.

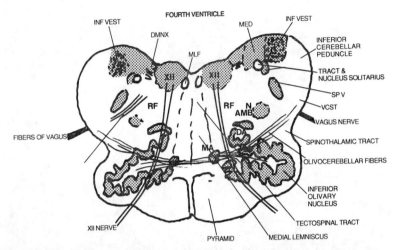

FIGURE 76. Brain stem section at the upper medulla; see Figure 73.

DA = dorsal accessory olivary nucleus; DMNX = dorsal motor nucleus of the vagus; INF VEST = inferior (spinal) vestibular nucleus including descending fibers of the lateral vestibulospinal tract; MA = medial accessory olivary nucleus; MED = medial vestibular nucleus; MLF = medial longitudinal fasciculus; N AMB = nucleus ambiguus (motor to pharynx and larynx); RF = reticular formation; SP V = spinal nucleus of the trigeminal (just lateral to the nucleus is the spinal tract); VCST = ventral spinocerebellar tract; XII = hypoglossal nucleus

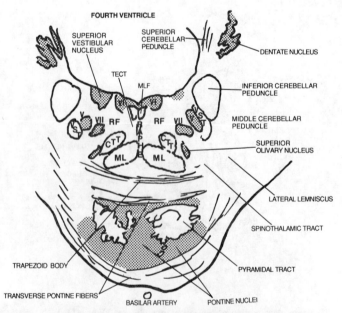

FIGURE 77. Brain stem section at lower pons; see Figure 73.

CTT = central tegmental tract; ML = medial lemniscus; MLF = medial longitudinal lemniscus; RF = reticular formation; TECT = tectobulbar and tectospinal tracts; V = spinal nucleus of trigeminal; VI = abducens nucleus; VII = facial nucleus; VST = spinal tract of trigeminal.

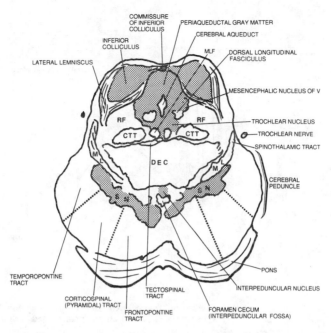

FIGURE 78. Brain stem section at the inferior colliculus; see Figure 73.
CTT = central tegmental tract; DEC = decussation of the superior cerebellar peduncle (brachium conjunctivum); ML = medial lemniscus; MLF = medial longitudinal fasciculus; RF = reticular formation; SN = substantia nigra.

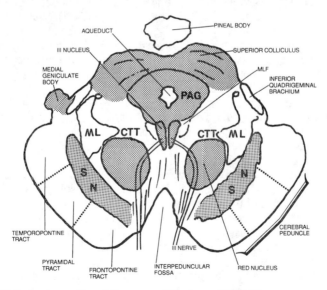

FIGURE 79. Brain stem section at the upper midbrain; see Figure 73.
CTT = central tegmental tract; ML = medial lemniscus; MLF = medial longitudinal fasciculus; PAG = periaqueductal gray; SN = substantia nigra.

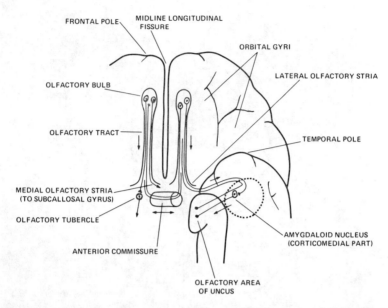

FIGURE 80. Projections of the olfactory bulb, as viewed from below. Only the fibers from olfactory bulb to uncus via lateral olfactory stria and amygdaloid nucleus are olfactory in function. (Correlate with Figures 4 and 124).

FACIAL NERVE (VII)

About 10,000 fibers make up the facial nerve, which also has several components. Most obvious are the fibers controlling muscles of facial expression, which arise from the facial nucleus (Figure 73). This nucleus also innervates the stapedius muscle (see Figure 103). The facial nerve exits from the cerebellopontine angle immediately ventral to the VIII nerve (Figures 4 and 96) and enters the internal auditory meatus with the VIII nerve. After a complex course through the petrous bone, it leaves the base of the skull via the stylomastoid foramen just medial to the mastoid process.

It also carried gustatory fibers from about 6000 taste buds in the anterior two-thirds of the tongue via the chorda tympani, and the nervus intermedius which lies in the cerebellopontine angle between VII and VIII nerves. First-order neurons for these sensory fibers form the geniculate ganglion which lies in the depths of the petrous bone.

Chorda tympani gets its name from its crossing the inner surface of the eardrum, the tympanum. Taste fibers terminate in the solitary nucleus of the medulla. Their upward projection path is uncertain, but taste appears to reach the cortex in the lower part of the parietal lobe near the face area.

Visceromotor parasympathetic fibers also travel in the nervus intermedius and chorda tympani to innervate submandibular and sublingual salivary glands, and via the greater superficial petrosal nerve to supply the lacrimal gland in the lateral corner of the orbit. These preganglionic axons arise from the salivatory

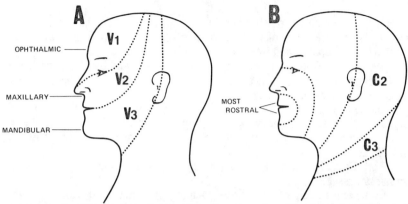

FIGURE 81. (A) Peripheral distribution of the three branches of the trigeminal (fifth cranial) nerve. (B) Segmental dermatomal pattern of facial sensory innervation. Note that the two patterns do not correspond, and that the perioral region is the most rostral part of the skin's sensory innervation.

nucleus at the rostral end of the dorsal motor nucleus of the vagus (Figures 73 and 137).

Facial paralysis most often results from lesions of the facial nerve. If due to a lower motor neuron lesion, Bell's palsy or other peripheral damage, the entire ipsilateral face will be paralyzed. Upper motor neuron lesions usually spare the forehead, because the part of the facial nucleus controlling forehead muscles receives bilateral cortical inputs.

VESTIBULOCOCHLEAR NERVE (VIII)

See Chapter 10.

GLOSSOPHARYNGEAL AND VAGUS NERVES (IX, X)

These two nerves are commonly considered together because of their overlapping functions. Nucleus ambiguus in the depths of the medulla (Figure 73) innervates volitional muscles of the pharynx by way of both ninth and tenth nerves, and the larynx via the vagus (for phonation). Larynx and pharynx have bilateral cortical (upper motor neuron) innervation, similar to the forehead. Unilateral cerebral lesions such as tumor or CVA do not usually cause paralysis of the forehead, or of phonation or deglutition. Of course, a lower motor neuron lesion (of the nerves themselves) will do so. Such paralysis is labeled bulbar palsy, bulb referring to medulla plus pons. Pseudobulbar palsy means paralysis of swallowing and phonation as a result of *bilateral* upper motor neuron lesions.

Glossopharyngeal and vagus lie in the cerebellopontine angle with VII and VIII and exit from the cranial cavity via the jugular foramen (Figures 3 and 96).

Sensation from the larynx enters the medulla via the vagus to terminate in nucleus solitarius. The same central connection for sensation from posterior pharynx mediates gag and cough reflexes. Pain sensibility for these regions enters with either nerve to terminate in the nucleus of the spinal tract of the trigeminal. Sensory fibers of each of the two nerves have their first-order cell bodies in small superior and inferior ganglia (Figure 96).

Taste fibers from posterior tongue travel via IX, and the vagus carries a few fibers from taste buds on the epiglottis. They terminate in the gustatory rostral part of the nucleus solitarius.

Glossopharyngeal secretomotor fibers supply the parotid salivary gland, originating from the salivatory nucleus (Figures 73 and 137), with a relay in the otic ganglion, which lies just outside the foramen ovale on the base of the skull (Figure 3).

Both IX and X innervate small mucus glands in lining of pharynx and respiratory passages.

Both nerves take part in cardiovascular and pulmonary reflexes, as already mentioned. Afferent inputs may be by way of either; effector fibers arising in the dorsal motor nucleus of the vagus mostly exit with the vagus, descending to the heart, lungs, and abdominal viscera.

ACCESSORY NERVE (XI)

A small nerve of about 3500 motor fibers, the accessory arises from upper cervical and lower medullary anterior horn cells, and supplies the sternomastoid and trapezius muscles. It also exits the cranial cavity via jugular foramen.

HYPOGLOSSAL NERVE (XII)

The hypoglossal nucleus forms a small ridge next to the midline in the posterior floor of the fourth ventricle (Figures 73, 76, and 97). Hypoglossal nerve fibers pass ventrally through inferior olivary nucleus to exit between pyramid and olive (Figure 4) and leave the cranial cavity via the anterior condylar (hypoglossal) foramen (Figure 3). It supplies striated muscles of the ipsilateral tongue.

CLINICAL EXAMPLE 21

A patient in his seventies suffered a CVA, with resultant left hemiplegia. He had no difficulty with speech, swallowing, phonation, or wrinkling his forehead.

Discussion

This left upper motor neuron hemiplegia probably resulted from a CVA in the internal capsule. Left-side spasticity and Babinski would be expected. Tongue, pharynx, and larynx as well as forehead were unaffected, undoubtedly because of bilateral cortical (UMN) innervation by cranial nerves VII, IX, X, and XII.

The tongue's bilateral innervation is somewhat unusual.

CLINICAL EXAMPLE 22

An elderly man had had numerous 'minor strokes' over the preceding three years. On examination, he was unable to frown or close his eyes tightly, and his gag reflex was absent bilaterally even though

*he felt the tongue blade uncomfortably in his throat. Discuss
these findings.*

Discussion

*Multiple vascular lesions of the cerebrum often damage motor
cortex or its projections bilaterally. As a result, motor functions of
facial (VII), glossopharyngeal (IX), and vagus (X) nerves become
weak (palsied). Because of the bilateral UMN input into these
motor cranial nerves, weakness (so-called 'bulbar palsy') is expected
only with damage to the nerves themselves or their nuclei. In
this patient, the bilateral UMN lesions led to bilateral weakness
of forehead and pharynx, often called 'pseudobulbar palsy' because of
its superficial similarity to bulbar palsy.*

CLINICAL EXAMPLE 23

*A woman gradually developed complete paralysis of the left face, lost
the ability to move her left eye laterally, lost much of the sensation
over the right half of her body, below the head, and then developed a
right spastic hemiplegia. Where was the lesion?*

Discussion

*Complete paralysis of the left face indicates a lesion in the left
facial nucleus or nerve, i.e., a peripheral facial palsy. Loss of
sensation over the right half of the body suggests a lesion in the
left medial lemniscus, left thalamus, or left internal capsule.
Neither spinal cord nor cortical lesions could do this. Why? Inability to
deviate the left eye laterally suggests a left VI palsy. Right
spastic hemiplegia suggests a lesion in the pyramidal tract, left
side, between foramen magnum and internal capsule. Again, neither
cord nor cortical lesion would be likely to do this. A single small lesion
in the left pons would account for all these findings. Gradual
development of the signs suggests a slowly growing tumor in the pons.
This combination of left facial and right arm-leg paralysis is called
alternating hemiplegia*

CLINICAL EXAMPLE 24

*A lady with known heart disease (atrial fibrillation) suddenly developed
a left hemiplegia, with paralysis of left arm and leg, and when asked
to stick out her tongue, it deviated to the right. Where was the lesion?*

Discussion

*With atrial fibrillation, small thrombi from the heart commonly travel
to the cerebral circulation to block small arteries. In this patient,
the blocked artery supplied the right ventral quadrant of the medulla at
the level where the right hypoglossal nerve exits between the
pyramid and the olive (see Figures 4, 75, and 76). Thus she
exhibited right-sided lower motor neuron paralysis of the tongue due
to damage to the right XII nerve, and a left-sided UMN paralysis of*

the arm and leg due to damage to the right pyramid, an alternating hemiplegia. Note that the absence of facial paralysis suggests that the lesion was caudal *to the facial nucleus and nerve (Figures 73, 77, and 96).*

CLINICAL EXAMPLE 25

A chronic smoker developed lung cancer, and just before beginning treatment noted numbness of the left side of her face. A few days later tingling began in her right shoulder which progressed to complete numbness of the entire right side of her body. On examination, the 'numbness' appeared to consist mostly of inability to recognize pin-prick stimulation or to detect warmth or cold. Proprioceptive sensibility and touch were essentially unimpaired.

Discussion

This 'alternating sensory loss' of pain and temperature sensory functions of the left side of the face and right side of the body can best be explained by a single lesion of the left lateral medulla. Damage to the descending spinal tract of the trigeminal caused the left facial sensory loss, and damage to the nearby spinothalamic tract caused the right-sided loss of pain and temperature sensation below the neck. In this patient, the damage undoubtedly resulted from a small growing metastasis of the lung cancer to the left lateral medulla. Review Figures 73-76.

Note that proprioceptive sensibility and touch, mostly carried in the paramedian medial lemniscus, were not disturbed.

CLINICAL EXAMPLE 26

A young man riding in the passenger seat without his seat belt was slammed against the windshield when the car rammed another car at about 40 km/hour. He remained unconscious for several hours. As he recovered alertness he complained of a copious discharge of watery fluid from his right nostril (rhinorrhea) and, when he could be tested, loss of the sense of smell in the right nostril (anosmia). The fluid had the chemical characteristics of cerebrospinal fluid. Explain these findings.

Discussion

At 40 km/hour, a head hitting a windshield is likely to be fractured. In this instance, the thin, fragile right cribriform plate (see Figure 3) was fractured, opening a passageway for the escape of CSF from the frontal subarachnoid space into the nasal cavity. The same fracture ruptured the olfactory nerve fibers on that side, causing the anosmia. The opening sometimes heals spontaneously. If not, it must be closed surgically to prevent infectious meningitis due to the entrance of bacteria from the nasal cavity into CSF spaces.

STUDY QUESTIONS

1. What is bulbar palsy?
2. What is pseudobulbar palsy?
3. What would you expect to find on examining a patient whose left uncus was destroyed by a CVA?
4. Clinical Examples 23 and 24 are crossed or alternating hemiplegias. What does this term mean?
5. PICA (the posterior inferior cerebellar artery) supplies blood to the lateral one-third of the medulla. What signs would you expect to follow occlusion of the left PICA? This is called a lateral medullary syndrome. (Study Figure 76.)
6. Account for the early loss of the corneal reflex and of facial sensation ipsilaterally as a cerebellopontine angle tumor develops.
7. What is the principal sign of an isolated lesion interrupting the right vagus nerve in the upper neck?
8. Review the clinical findings associated with unilateral lesions of each of the cranial nerves.

9 Visual Systems

Vision far exceeds in importance all other sensory modalities in human experience. The cortical areas for vision are large and complex, the motor correlates of visual function include anatomical structures extending from cortex to cervical spinal cord, and numerous reflex systems control important aspects of voluntary and automatic visual behavior.

THE EYE

The eye (bulb, eyeball, bulbus oculi) is a sphere about 22 mm in diameter lying in the anterior part of the bony orbit, held in place by muscular attachments, optic nerve, orbital fat pads, conjunctiva, and eyelids. Within the constraints of the surrounding structures, the bulb rotates freely in any direction, much like a ball bearing.

Light enters the eye through the cornea, which does most of the refracting, proceeds inward through aqueous humor and lens, which acts to vary refraction, and through the vitreous humor to impinge on the retina with its light-sensitive rods and cones.

In normal eyes at rest, parallel rays of light, that is, rays from an object at infinite distance, are focused on the retina. To focus nearby objects, the lens becomes more convex, rounding up under its own elasticity, when the ciliary muscle (Figure 82) contracts to release some of the radial tension on the lens. As age increases, the lens hardens and loses its elasticity, so that focusing nearby objects becomes impossible. This is farsightedness, hypermetropia or hyperopia of elderly individuals; also called presbyopia (Greek = old-age vision). Myopia, or nearsightedness, refers to the inability to focus on distant objects (Figure 83).

Astigmatism occurs when the cornea is not spherical, and so has greater curvature in one meridian than another. As a result, focusing is good in one meridian, poor in another. More rarely, the cornea may be congenitally distorted in other ways, such as keratoconus where it is cone shaped,, and focusing is impossible. These refractive problems can usually be corrected with lenses of various types.

The cornea and sclera form the tough wall of the globe. Just inside the white sclera is the choroid, a vascular layer, and inside this lies the retina lining the posterior two-thirds of the eye. The space behind the lens is filled with clear, vitreous humor.

Aqueous humor, filling the anterior chamber, is similar to CSF (cerebrospinal fluid), and, like CSF, may develop increased pressure, usually due to obstruction of its drainage into the canal of Schlemm. Increased intraocular pressure can cut off blood supply to the retina and cause blindness. This condition is called glaucoma.

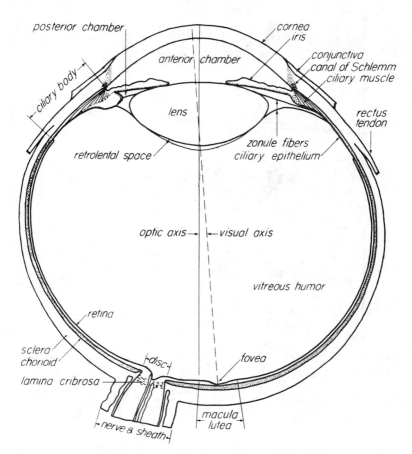

FIGURE 82. Horizontal section of right human eye. The optic nerve sheath is continuous with cranial dura. Aqueous humor, formed in the posterior chamber, flows through the pupil into the anterior chamber and is resorbed into the venous canal of Schlemm. (Courtesy of Cranbrook Institute of Science.)

Blood supply to the retina comes by way of two systems. Just behind (outside) the retinal layer is the choroid or chorioid (see Figure 82), a layer of small blood vessels. In front of the retina, between it and the vitreous humor lie the retinal vessels, which can be seen through the pupil with an ophthalmoscope. Neither system actually penetrates the retinal layer, so that nutritive substances and oxygen must get to retinal cells by diffusion. Both systems appear to be necessary for normal retinal function.

THE RETINA

Embryologically, the light-sensitive retina develops from the diencephalon as an extension of the CNS. Glia is present in the adult retina just as in the CNS, and subarachnoid space surrounds the optic nerve all the way out to the bulb. The retina can be examined through the pupil using an ophthalmo-

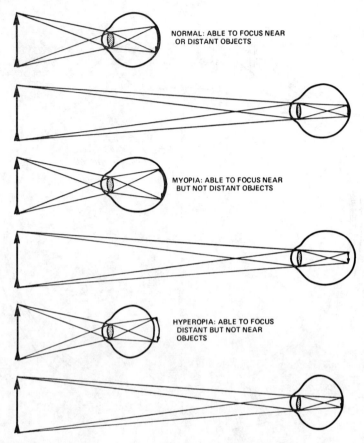

FIGURE 83. Note that the ocular chamber is relatively too long with myopia (middle two diagrams), and too short with hyperopia (lower two diagrams). Note also the inversion of images.

scope. Retinal blood vessels can be examined directly to detect arteriosclerosis and other abnormalities. Changes in the optic disc such as papilledema or pallor from atrophy may also be detected.

Papilledema (choked disc, swelling of the optic disc) may result from increased intracranial pressure, acting at the attachment of optic nerve to bulb, where the increased CSF pressure compresses veins draining the retina to cause local edema.

In mammals, the retina consists of layered cells, processes and terminals (Figure 84). The retinal layer next to the choroid is the pigment epithelium which phagocytoses degenerated visual pigments from rods and cones. Rods and cones synapse with bipolar cells, which in turn synapse with retinal ganglion cells, whose axons exit via the optic disc to form the optic nerve. Horizontal and amacrine cells (Figure 84) are interneurons concerned with definition of edges.

The human retina consists of about 120 million rods and 6 million cones. In a small macular area at the center of the retina, the region of acute, high resolution vision, is a small depression called the fovea (Latin = pit), where only close-packed cones exist (Figure 82). Here each cone projects to one ganglion cell, mediating high resolution. In the peripheral retina, there are more rods than cones, and many rods project to a single ganglion cell, mediating high light sensitivity but poor resolution.

Sensitivity of the human retina extends over a tremendous range. The intensity of bright sunlight on clean snow is about 10^{10} (ten billion) times as great as the dimness of a moonless night, yet both extremes can be seen by properly-adapted normal eyes.

Scotopic or night vision has been attributed to rods, and photopic or day-time vision to cones. Photopic vision is best in the macular area, where scotopic vision does not occur. Scotopic vision is best in the paramacular (para-foveal) region, where the number of rods is maximum. Because of this distribution of rods, dim stars or other night objects are best seen by looking slightly to one side rather than directly at them.

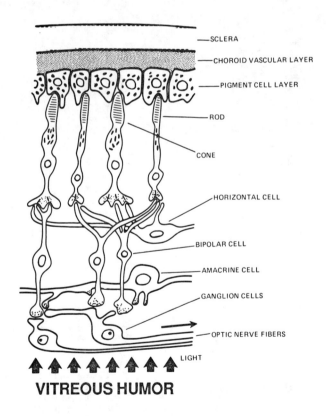

VITREOUS HUMOR

FIGURE 84. Pattern of retinal layers. (Simplified after Dowling and Boycott: Proc. Roy. Soc. (B), 166:80-111, 1966.)

The mechanism of color vision remains incompletely understood, despite 200 years of study. Cones contain visual pigments (chromophores) of three different wavelength sensitivities: 445 millimicrons (blue), 535 millimicrons (green), and 570 millimicrons (red); rods contain rhodopsin, maximally sensitive at 505 millimicrons. Interactions between cones (and possibly rods) with these various pigments accounts for our ability to distinguish up to one million shades of color, but no one knows how this occurs.

Individual rods or cones consist of the usual cytologic components, with the addition of a light-sensitive external segment, which appears to be a modified cilium, and contains about 1000 flattened saccules (laminae; Figure 85) to which are attached about 10,000,000 molecules of rhodopsin (rods) or other chromophores (cones).

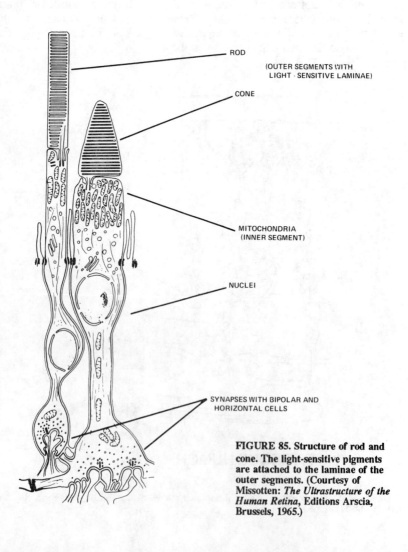

ROD

(OUTER SEGMENTS WITH LIGHT - SENSITIVE LAMINAE)

CONE

MITOCHONDRIA (INNER SEGMENT)

NUCLEI

SYNAPSES WITH BIPOLAR AND HORIZONTAL CELLS

FIGURE 85. Structure of rod and cone. The light-sensitive pigments are attached to the laminae of the outer segments. (Courtesy of Missotten: *The Ultrastructure of the Human Retina*, Editions Arscia, Brussels, 1965.)

When rods or cones are at rest, a constant dark current flows from the inner segment to the outer segment, giving the retina a constant positive potential with respect to the back of the eye. This can be measured at the cornea. Light striking the cell causes sudden hyperpolarization of the outer segment, probably calcium-mediated.

This potential change acts through bipolar cells to induce action potentials in ganglion cells. Rods, cones, horizontal cells, and amacrine cells respond in graded fashion; the first action potentials are generated in ganglion cells.

The complex series of graded potentials generated in the retina can be recorded at the cornea as the electroretinogram (ERG).

CLINICAL EXAMPLE 27

A 25-year-old man came to the physician's office because of increasing difficulty with vision. No abnormalities were found except for decreased visual acuity 20/200 OS (left eye) and 20/300 OD (right eye). His visual fields showed a punched out scotoma or blind spot covering the macular area of each eye. The working diagnosis was macular degeneration, cause unknown.

Explain the visual difficulties brought on by macular degeneration, when the rest of the retina is normal. Would you expect this patient to see better in daylight or at night?

Discussion

Scotomas in macular areas destroy acute vision, accounting for the patient's very poor visual acuity. Inasmuch as his peripheral retina remains normal, you might expect him to have normal scotopic (night) vision, but poor daytime vision.

VISUAL PATHWAYS

Central pathways for vision (Figure 86) begin with type 'X' retinal ganglion cells whose myelinated axons exit from the bulb through the optic disc to form the optic nerve. The 1 million fibers of the optic nerve extend back to the optic chiasm, where about 50 percent decussate, joining the undecussated 50 percent from the other retina to form the optic tract. Each optic tract proceeds back around the base of the cerebral peduncle to the lateral geniculate body (LGB) of the thalamus, where the first extraretinal synapse occurs.

Three of the layers of the six-layered lateral geniculate receive axon terminals from the contralateral hemifield of the contralateral eye, the other three layers from the contralateral hemifield of the ipsilateral eye. Though these inputs from the two eyes lie adjacent to each other, the neurons do not interact— binocular vision is not mediated in the LGB.

Next-order axons from LGB sweep backward in the deep white matter of temporal, parietal, and occipital lobes as the geniculocalcarine or optic radiation. These fibers form the external sagittal stratum (Figure 91), and are separated from the lateral ventricle by the internal sagittal stratum (descending fibers from area 18, Figure 93), and by the tapetum, fibers of the corpus callosum on the ventricular surface. Most of the fibers terminate in cortical layer 4 of the

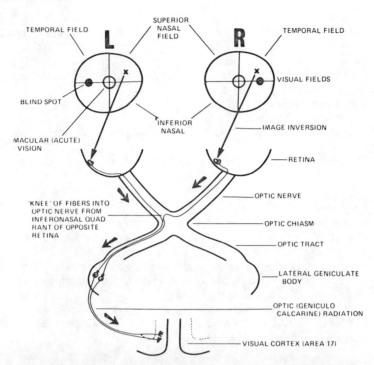

TEMPORAL FIELD

SUPERIOR NASAL FIELD

TEMPORAL FIELD

VISUAL FIELDS

BLIND SPOT

INFERIOR NASAL

IMAGE INVERSION

MACULAR (ACUTE) VISION

RETINA

'KNEE' OF FIBERS INTO OPTIC NERVE FROM INFERONASAL QUADRANT OF OPPOSITE RETINA

OPTIC NERVE

OPTIC CHIASM

OPTIC TRACT

LATERAL GENICULATE BODY

OPTIC (GENICULO CALCARINE) RADIATION

VISUAL CORTEX (AREA 17)

FIGURE 86. Visual pathway. X in the right superior visual quadrants represent a single object in front of the subject. Note that right and left half-fields project to the contralateral visual cortices. Hemidecussation in the chiasm brings together fibers from visually corresponding points in the right and left retinas, related to corresponding images in the visual fields of right and left eye. This provides the basis for binocular vision.

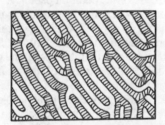

FIGURE 87. Ocular dominance pattern in the visual cortex of a monkey. Dark strips receive visual projections from the ipsilateral eye, light strips from the contralateral eye. Each strip is about 0.5 mm wide.

upper and lower lip of the calcarine fissure on the medial aspect of the occipital lobe. Inputs from the two eyes project to adjacent strips of the visual cortex as 'ocular dominance columns' about 0.5 mm across. The entire visual cortex thus shows a pattern of strips alternately projecting from ipsilateral and from contralateral eye (Figure 87). Neuronal interactions between these adjacent strips or columns of cortex mediate binocular vision.

Visual cortex has several synonyms: calcarine cortex, area 17 of Brodmann, striate cortex (because of the stria of Gennari, a heavy lamina of myelinated fibers in layer 4).

VISUAL FIELDS

Clinical examination of visual pathways consists first of careful evaluation of the visual fields. The visual field of each eye must be studied separately. Because we possess binocular vision, the visual fields of right and left eye would have identical fields of view except that the nose blocks part of the medial or nasal part of the visual field of each eye.

Each visual field is divided into nasal and temporal half-fields, and into superior and inferior half-fields; thus into four quadrants; superior nasal, superior temporal, inferior nasal, and inferior temporal (Figure 86).

A physiological blind spot to the temporal side of the macular area in each visual field corresponds to the optic disc (Figures 82 and 86) which has no rods or cones.

Figures 88 and 89 show visual field losses resulting from common lesions of the visual pathways. Note that lesions in front of the chiasm always cause visual field loss in one eye, while lesions behind the chiasm always cause visual field losses in both eyes, more or less similar (congruent). When evaluating partial lesions of the visual pathways, it is useful to recall that the farther back the lesion, i.e., the closer to the cortex, the more nearly congruent the field defects in the two eyes: a small cortical lesion causes identical scotomas in the visual fields of right and left eyes.

Total destruction of any of the structures making up the visual pathway behind the chiasm on one side causes a contralateral homonymous hemianopia (Figure 88B or C). CVAs resulting from occlusion of the posterior cerebral artery frequently cause contralateral homonymous hemianopia (Figures 21 and 88) because this artery supplies the entire occipital lobe. Effects of chiasmatic lesions are more complex (Figure 89).

To complete a gross description of the visual pathways, they must also be viewed from the side (Figure 90). Impulses from the upper retina project via the upper fibers of the optic radiation, deep to the parietal cortex, to terminate in the upper lip of the calcarine fissure. Lower retinal impulses project to the lower lip of the calcarine fissure via fibers sweeping down into the temporal lobe. Because they swing laterally to go around the lateral ventricle (Figure 91), the optic radiations lie close to the cortex, and may be damaged by cortical lesions, as in Figure 90. Because the fibers fan out widely, a lesion often will damage only a portion of them, leading to homonymous scotomas or to homonymous quadrantic visual field defects.

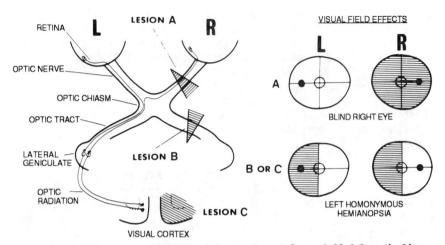

FIGURE 88. Effects of complete lesions of visual pathway before or behind the optic chiasm.

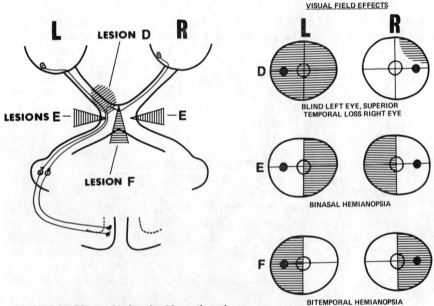

FIGURE 89. Effects of lesions in chiasmatic region.
   D = Damage to optic nerve and to the loop of fibers from the in-
         ferior nasal retina of the other eye.
   E = Rare; requires bilaterally symmetrical lesions. Most likely
         due to bilateral internal carotid aneurysms. (Review circle of
         Willis, Figures 16 and 17.)
   F = Midchiasmatic lesion most commonly caused by pituitary
         tumor.

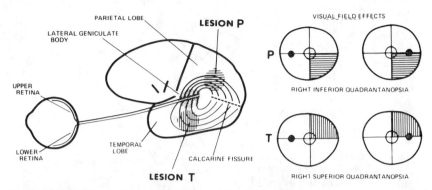

FIGURE 90. Lesion P, interrupting optic radiation fibers from upper retina; and lesion T interrupting relay fibers from the lower retina, both cause contralateral quadrantic visual field defects.

MACULAR VISION

High-resolution or acute vision depends on the macular retina about the fovea (compare Clinical Example 27). Despite its relatively small area, the high density of cones there means that its projecting fibers make up a large portion of the optic nerve, and it projects to about two-thirds of the visual cortex. The macular cortex lies most occipital; the rostral one-third of the calcarine cortex receives inputs from peripheral vision (see Figure 2).

Clinically, the large area of the macular projection means that a large lesion is needed to destroy it. This has the interesting effect that a lesion causing a hemianopia as determined by evaluating peripheral fields may leave a large portion of macular function intact. The term macular sparing has been applied to this phenomenon.

PUPILLARY LIGHT REFLEXES

When a bright light is shone into one eye, both pupils constrict reflexly. This pupillary light reflex protects the retina from bright lights. The afferent pathway for the reflex follows that for vision as far as the lateral geniculate body (Figure 92), but along the axons of a different set of retinal ganglion cells ('W' cells) than those ('X' cells) concerned with vision. The reflex axons bypass the lateral geniculate without synapsing, to end in the pretectal nucleus, a small collection of neurons immediately rostral to the superior colliculus.

Next-order fibers loop around the periaqueductal gray of the midbrain, either directly to the oculomotor (III) nucleus of the same side, or to the oculo-motor nucleus of the opposite side via the decussation in the posterior com-missure. They synapse with parasympathetic neurons in the oculomotor nucleus whose efferent axons exit with the III nerve. Most of these fibers synapse in the ciliary ganglion just behind the eye, whence postganglionic fibers continue into the eye as the ciliary nerves to innervate the smooth circular constrictor muscle of the iris (Figure 92).

Note in Figure 92 that two decussations, in optic chiasm and in posterior commissure, insure that both pupils will constrict if one eye is stimulated. Constriction (miosis) of the directly stimulated eye is called the direct light reflex; constriction of the other pupil, the consensual reflex.

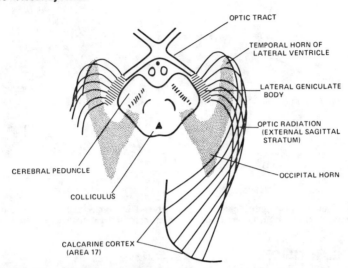

FIGURE 91. Horizontal view of relationship between optic radiation and temporal and occipital horns of the lateral ventricle.

Parasympathetic fibers cause constriction (miosis) of the pupil. Dilation (mydriasis) results from activity of sympathetic fibers. These pupillodilator impulses originate in the ipsilateral hypothalamus, descending by way of long fibers through the brain stem and cervical cord to the first and second thoracic segments (T 1-2). There they synapse with ipsilateral sympathetic neurons, whose axons exit as preganglionic fibers, and ascend the sympathetic chain in the neck to synapse in the superior cervical ganglion. Postganglionic fibers form a plexus around the internal carotid artery, thence by various routes into the orbit, eventually to innervate the radial smooth dilator muscle of the iris (Figure 137).

Horner's syndrome, the result of a lesion in this sympathetic pathway, appears clinically as a constantly miotic pupil, often associated with anhidrosis (lack of sweating) of the forehead, and usually ptosis of the upper lid on the same side. It is important to recognize that Horner's syndrome may result from lesions of sympathetic fibers either inside or outside the CNS.

ACCOMMODATION REFLEXES — Near Reflex

To fixate a nearby object visually, three reflex changes occur, which make up the accommodation or near reflex: (1) Miosis — pupilloconstriction. (2) Lenticular accommodation — resulting from contraction of the ciliary muscle to diminish the circumferential tension on the lens, thus focusing on nearby objects (see Figure 82 and 83 and page 96). (3) Convergence of the visual axes through contraction of the medial rectus muscles.

Visual impulses arrive at area 17 in the usual way (Figures 86 and 93). From there impulses pass to the adjacent parastriate cortex, area 18, from which fibers descend in the internal sagittal stratum of occipital white matter to the region of the superior colliculus and pretectal area. There impulses are relayed to parasympathetic neurons of the III nerves, and to the nuclei for

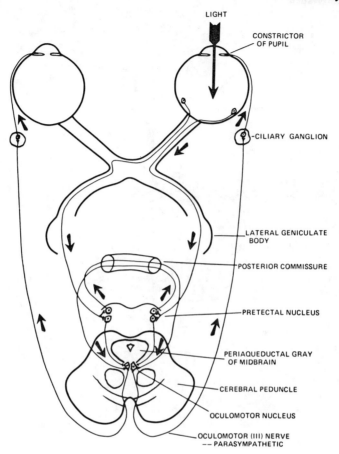

LIGHT

CONSTRICTOR OF PUPIL

CILIARY GANGLION

LATERAL GENICULATE BODY

POSTERIOR COMMISSURE

PRETECTAL NUCLEUS

PERIAQUEDUCTAL GRAY OF MIDBRAIN

CEREBRAL PEDUNCLE

OCULOMOTOR NUCLEUS

OCULOMOTOR (III) NERVE
-- PARASYMPATHETIC

FIGURE 92. Pathways for the pupillary light reflex.

medial rectus muscles, and finally to the eye to cause contraction of pupillo-constrictor, ciliary, and medial rectus muscles.

LIGHT - NEAR DISSOCIATION: The Argyll Robertson Pupil

Lack of pupillary light reflex with normal accommodation (an intact near reflex) has been called Argyll Robertson pupil. Pupillary light reflex pathways must be damaged without damage to accommodation pathways: this may occur in the periaqueductal gray, where accommodation fibers travel more ventrally than light reflex fibers, or in the ciliary ganglion, where there are 30 times as many accommodation as light-responding fibers. Compare Figure 93. The Argyll Robertson pupil used to be considered pathognomonic for CNS lues. With the relative rarity of untreated syphilis nowadays, other kinds of small vessel disease, such as diabetes, arteriosclerosis, or systemic lupus erythematosus are more likely.

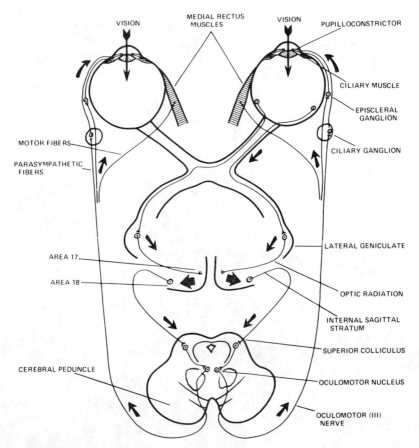

FIGURE 93. Pathways for the accommodation reflexes: (1) pupilloconstriction; (2) lenticular focusing by contraction of ciliary muscles; and (3) convergence by contraction of medial rectus muscles.

CLINICAL EXAMPLE 28

A diabetic gentleman, age 55, was seen because of visual difficulties. His diabetes was under good control, and he had no apparent retinal damage from the disease, except for mild arteriosclerosis. His pupils were almost unreactive: the right pupil constricted very slightly, the left not at all to bright light. Both constricted well when he fixated a nearby object, i.e., accommodation reflexes were normal. Where is the lesion?

Discussion

These are bilateral Argyll Robertson pupils. From the discussion above, you may conclude that the lesion is either in the periaqueductal gray or in the ciliary ganglia.

EXTRAOCULAR MUSCLES

As suggested by Figure 94, movements of the visual axis, i.e., movements of the direction of gaze, result from contraction of one or more of the six extraocular muscles; lateral, medial, superior and inferior rectus, and superior and inferior obliques. The seventh muscle, the levator palpebrae, elevates the upper lid.

CONJUGATE EYE MOVEMENTS: BRAIN STEM MECHANISMS

All normal movements of the eyes for observing an object in visual space are conjugate: both eyes always move simultaneously to fixate and focus on a single point for binocular vision. It is, in fact, impossible for a normal individual to move one eye at a time voluntarily. The demonstrations of apparent monocular movements require that one eye be so positioned that it is already fixated on a terminal fixation point, so that only the other eye needs to move.

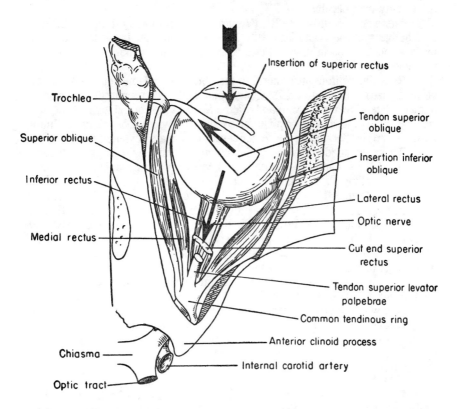

FIGURE 94. The extraocular muscles. Note that the superior rectus muscle (arrowhead) pulls at an angle 20 degrees lateral to the visual axis (complete arrow), and that the superior oblique (arrowhead) pulls 40 degrees medial to the visual axis. (Modified and reproduced, with permission from Peele: *The Neuroanatomical Basis for Clinical Neurology*, McGraw-Hill, New York, 1977.)

Moreover, all 12 of the muscles of both eyes contract or are inhibited from contraction simultaneously in nearly all eye movements. The accuracy of these multiple simultaneous contractions is astounding.

To permit such supremely accurate conjugate movements, the 12 extra-ocular muscles, their six cranial nerves and nuclei, and the medial longitudinal fasciculus (MLF) operate as a unit. The MLF interconnects cranial nerve nuclei III, IV, and VI, as well as cervical anterior horn cells concerned with head movements. So long as this complex remains intact and normally functional, all eye movements remain conjugate. A lesion anywhere in the complex (muscles, nerves, nuclei, or MLF) will disrupt conjugate gaze, and the patient will usually complain of diplopia or double vision. Refer to Figures 94 and 98.

HIGHER LEVEL CONTROL OF EYE MOVEMENTS

Control of the brain stem oculomotor mechanisms resides in several centers: (1) Pontine gaze center (PGC) in the reticular formation of the pontine tegmentum next to the VI nerve nucleus. (2) Subtectal and pretectal centers next to the superior colliculus. (3) Vestibular nuclei. (4) Cerebellum, particularly the flocculus.

These centers influence III, IV, and VI nuclei directly through MLF and tectobulbar pathways, and indirectly by way of the reticular formation of the brain stem. Lesions in any of these places may have striking effects on eye movements.

Reticular neurons just lateral to the abducens (VI) nucleus make up the pontine gaze center (Figure 95). Their axonal outflow goes into the adjacent VI nucleus (lateral rectus muscle) and via the MLF to the contralateral III nucleus (medial rectus muscle) for ispilateral conjugate deviation of the eyes. Stimu-lation of the right pontine gaze center causes conjugate deviation of eyes to the right. These are sudden, saccadic, movements. Recent work suggests that the pontine gaze center and superior colliculus cooperate for saccadic movements.

Bilateral inputs from subtectal and pretectal neurons control up and down eye movement via MLF and tectobulbar fibers to III, IV, and VI. Each superior colliculus relates point-to-point to movements in the opposite visual field in experimental animals, and probably in humans. The rostromedial edge of each superior colliculus and adjacent pretectal neurons have to do with direct vertical eye movement (Figures 95 and 98). This region has been called the vertical gaze center (compare Clinical Example 29).

In response to position and movement of the head in space, vestibular nuclei send inputs to III, IV, and VI of both sides to induce eye movements consonant with the head movement. In normal individuals, this takes the form of vestibular nystagmus, with alternating saccades in the direction of head turning followed by slower smooth pursuit movement of the eyes in the opposite direction, to fix the eyes on an object. Vestibular connections through the pontine gaze center probably mediate the saccades; direct connections via MLF of both sides mediate the smooth pursuit movements (Figure 98).

Cerebellar connections into the oculomotor apparatus have been defined at the cellular level. They appear concerned with overall coordination of head and eye movements.

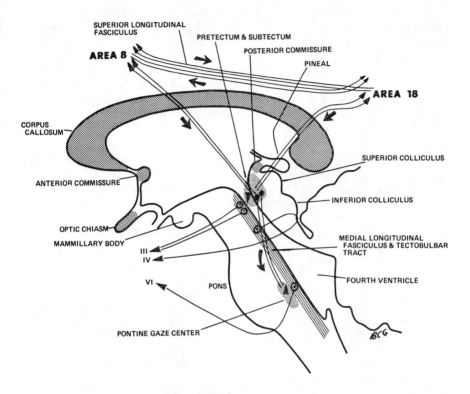

FIGURE 95. Structures involved in volitional eye movement. The superior longitudinal fasciculus is a large intracerebral bundle of fibers interconnecting cortical areas 8 and 18. The descending fibers from area 8 to the pontine gaze center are crossed; those from area 18 to the subtectum are bilateral.

HIGHEST LEVEL OF OCULOMOTOR CONTROL

Cortical mechanisms mediate volitional control of eye movements. Contralateral saccadic movements appear to be controlled by the frontal eye fields (area 8; area for adversive conjugate deviation; Figures 95 and 116). Microelectrode recording from this cortical region has revealed no action potentials prior to eye movements, a finding difficult to interpret. Area 8 projects, via corticobulbar fibers in the anterior limb of the internal capsule, to the pontine gaze center of the opposite side, mostly with relays in the superior colliculus. Lesions in area 8 or its connections may make it impossible for the patient to move the eyes volitionally to the opposite side. Such lesions in monkeys appear to cause 'neglect' of the opposite field of vision, which suggests that its function may be sensory rather than motor.

From the parastriate cortex of the occipital lobe (area 18), numerous fibers descend by a route similar to that for the accommodation reflexes (Figures 93 and 116), first in the internal sagittal stratum, then via the posterior limb of the internal capsule, to the subtectal and pretectal regions of both sides (Figures 95 and 98). This cortical connection appears to mediate smooth pursuit movements. Patients with occipital lesions may be unable to follow an object moving in the contralateral visual field, even though saccadic movements remain normal. A very large bundle of fibers, the superior longitudinal fasciculus (Fiugres 95 and 121) interconnects areas 8 and 18 and probably coordinates volitional oculomotor control.

CLINICAL EXAMPLE 29

A young woman visiting from India came to the hospital because of headaches and difficulty with vision. She had bilateral papilledema, and was unable to elevate her eyes above the horizontal. Diagnostic studies confirmed the presence of a pinealoma, a tumor of the pineal gland.

Discussion

Papilledema ordinarily results from increased intracranial (CSF) pressure. This patient's increased pressure resulted from compression of the cerebral aqueduct by the pinealoma (compare Figures 2, 28, and 97). Hydrocephalus then developed in lateral and third ventricles, associated with headaches. Inability to elevate the eyes resulted from damage to the vertical gaze center at the rostromedial edges of the superior colliculi.

CLINICAL EXAMPLE 30

Three months before she was seen, a 41-year-old lady had a convulsive seizure beginning with turning of her head to the right. An EEG (electroencephalogram) showed an abnormal spiking focus in the left midfrontal region. No tumor was found on careful study, so she was treated with anticonvulsants, and had no further seizures.

Discussion

Initiation of a convulsive seizure with turning of the eyes, head, and body suggests that the convulsive discharge probably began in or near the frontal eye field (area 8 — see Figures 95 and 116) of the side opposite the direction of turning (adversive). The EEG supported this interpretation.

MEDIAL LONGITUDINAL FASCICULUS (MLF)

From the posterior commissure, the MLF extends the full length of the brain stem, to upper cervical levels, Figures 95 and 98. Its major function is the control and coordination of eye movements. Visual motor inputs arise from vestibular nuclei, from the superior colliculus, and from the pontine gaze center. It also carries impulses from more rostral suprasegmental centers. Many MLF fibers interconnect nuclei III, IV, and VI of the two sides to make

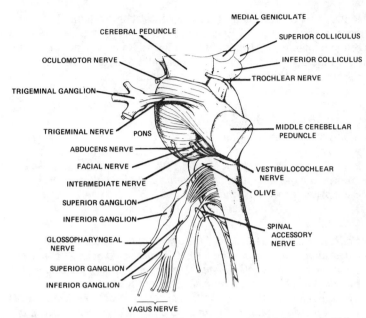

FIGURE 96. Brain stem and cranial nerves, lateral view (compare Figure 4). (Reproduced, with permission, from Truex and Carpenter: *Human Neuroanatomy, 6th ed.* Williams & Wilkins, Baltimore, 1969.)

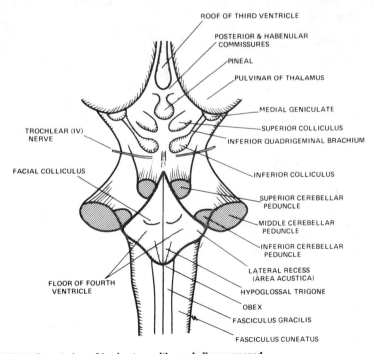

FIGURE 97. Dorsal view of brain stem with cerebellum removed.

possible the exact coordination of muscle contraction for normal conjugate eye movement (compare Clinical Example 31). It is one of the oldest of the long tracts of the human CNS. These observations reinforce the important primitive functions of the tract in maintenance of upright posture of the head, and adjustment of eyes and head in response to stimuli from eyes, from vestibular system, and from joint proprioceptors in the neck.

CLINICAL EXAMPLE 31

A 62-year-old man with an old, treated luetic infection was generally well except for problems in eye movement. The eye on the side toward which he attempted to gaze deviated irregularly, and the other eye would move only to midposition or perhaps a bit further. Other eye movements were normal.

Discussion

Conjugate lateral deviation of the eyes requires intact MLF connections between the abducens (VI) and oculomotor (III) nuclei, see Figure 98. Normally, impulses from the pontine gaze center feed into the VI nucleus to cause ipsilateral deviation of the ipsilateral eye through contraction of the lateral rectus muscle, and, via the MLF to the opposite III nucleus to innervate the medial rectus muscle of the other eye so it will deviate in the same direction. Thus, this gentleman's lesion, probably vascular, must be in the MLF between the VI and III nuclei. This syndrome is called internuclear ophthalmoplegia.

CLINICAL EXAMPLE 32

An elderly gentleman suffered a stroke. When he recovered conciousness, he was unable to move his left arm and leg, and the left side of his mouth drooped. He also complained bitterly about double vision. On examination, he had a left UMN paralysis, a left homonymous hemianopsia, and movements of his right eye were defective — lateral deviation was normal, and deviation downward and in was pretty good, but no other movements were possible. There was also no pupillary response to light. Where was the lesion?

Discussion

Left spastic hemiplegia suggests a pyramidal lesion on the right side above the medulla in view of the lower facial involvement. Left homonymous hemianopsia must result from a lesion of the visual pathway on the right side behind the chiasm, and the right ophthalmoplegia and lack of pupillary response indicate a lesion of the right oculomotor nerve. These three pathways lie close to each other in the midbrain region, and are commonly supplied by the posterior cerebral artery. Occlusion of this artery near its bifurcation from the basilar undoubtedly damaged the right cerebral peduncle, the right optic tract as it loops around the peduncle, and the right III nerve as it exits into the interpeduncular fossa. Review Figures 17, 20, 79, 88, and 92.

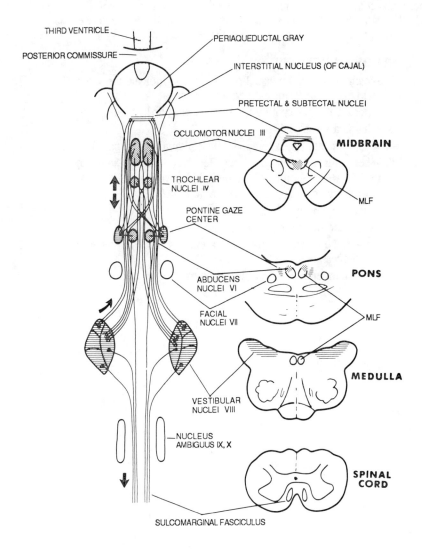

FIGURE 98. Medial longitudinal fasciculus (MLF); summary of connections and topography. MLF fibers descending to the cervical cord make up the sulcomarginal fasciculus, also called medial vestibulospinal fibers.

As discussed in the chapter on motor function, there is important functional overlap between proprioceptive inputs and pyramidal tract activity. Similarly, visual motor systems play an important and intrinsic role in the sensations of vision.

In summary, vision is our most important sensory input, emphasized by the complexity of the visual pathways themselves, by the large cortical areas mediating visual functions, by the elaborate mechanisms in cortex and brain stem for control of eye movements, and by the severe motor disturbances which result from lesions in the visual system. It has been well said that vision is our most important proprioceptive modality.

STUDY QUESTIONS

1. Sketch and label the visual pathways, and indicate the visual field effects of lesions at various levels.
2. Where is the ciliary muscle? What does it do?
3. What is a visual field?
4. What is meant by scotoma? — by diplopia? — by papilledema?
5. Where must a lesion be to cause left homonymous hemanopia?
6. What is the usual effect of stimulation of the left-sided eye field for adversive conjugate deviation (area 8)?
7. What is the normal blind spot?
8. Define the functions of the superior colliculus.
9. How is the medial longitudinal fasciculus (MLF) involved in the process of seeing?
10. Summarize the three levels of control of eye movement.

10 Vestibulocochlear Nerve

Two functionally distinct sensory divisions, the vestibular nerve and the cochlear nerve, make up the eighth cranial or vestibulocochlear nerve (old name acoustic). The former responds to position and movement of the head, subsuming functions often identified as equilibrium. The latter mediates auditory functions.

External structures associated with the eighth nerve are divided grossly into external ear, middle ear, and inner ear (Figure 99).

The external ear consists of the auricle (pinna, ear lobe), the external auditory meatus (canal), and the tympanum (eardrum).

AUDITORY MEATUS

Sound waves in the air enter the external auditory meatus and impinge on the tympanum, causing it to vibrate. Resonant frequency of the external and middle ear structures is 1000-2000 Hz (cycles per second), the frequency range of most human voices.

The vibration is transmitted through the air-filled middle ear cavity by way of three tiny bones, the ossicles: the malleus (hammer), the incus (anvil), and the stapes (stirrup). The malleus, attached to the inner aspect of the tympanum, transmits its vibration to the incus through a diarthrodial joint. Incus in turn articulates with stapes, which sits on the membrane of the foramen ovale (oval window), through which the vibration is transmitted to the fluid perilymph of the inner ear.

Mechanical transmission of vibration from the eardrum via the ossicles to the foramen ovale decreases the amplitude but increases the force of the vibration about 23-fold. The tympanic membrane is about 18 times as large as the foramen ovale, and the ossicles provide a mechanical advantage of 1.3 times: $1.3 \times 18 = 23$. This increased force of vibration makes it possible for sound vibration of air molecules to induce vibration in the fluid perilymph of the inner ear.

From the cavity of the middle ear to the posterior nasopharynx, the eustachian tube equalizes air pressures inside and outside the tympanic membrane. Also within the middle ear are two small muscles, the stapedius, innervated by the VII cranial nerve, and the tensor tympani, innervated by V cranial nerve. The stapedius muscle pulls on the stapes, the tensor tympani on the malleus, tightening the membranes respectively of the foramen ovale and of the tympanum, thereby decreasing the transmission of vibrational energy from outside to the inner ear.

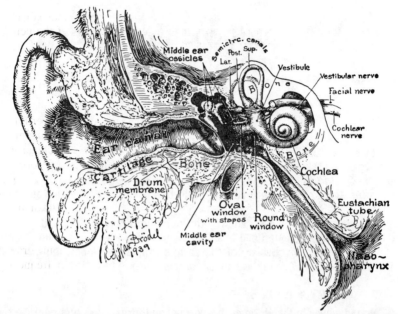

FIGURE 99. The gross anatomy of the external, middle, and internal ear. (After Brodel, courtesy of W. B. Saunders Company.)

CLINICAL EXAMPLE 33.

A 4-year-old brought in because of earache was obviously uncomfortable, had a fever of 102F (39C), and complained when his right ear was touched. The drum was red and inflamed, and dullness of the light reflex suggested inflammatory exudate (pus) in the middle ear. What would you expect to be the condition of the child's eustachian tube? Why is this important?

Discussion

Because of the inflammation of the middle ear (otitis media), the mucous lining of the eustachian tube swells, closing off the connection with the nasopharynx, and preventing equalization of pressures across the tympanic membrane. The closure also prevents the inflammatory exudate's draining out of the middle ear into the throat. If the pus is not drained, as by incising the tympanic membrane (myringotomy), the infection is likely to destroy the ossicles and other structures of the middle ear and cause permanent deafness. Such an incision will also relieve the pressure on the eardrum and with it much of the child's pain.

The inner ear consists of two major components corresponding to the two divisions of the VIII nerve: the cochlea (Latin = snail), which is the organ for hearing, and the vestibular apparatus, made up of three semicircular canals, a utricle, and a saccule. The entire complex is called the membranous labyrinth, contained within the cavity of the bony labyrinth in the depths of the petrous ridge of the temporal bone of the base of the skull. (Review Figure 3.)

COCHLEA

Resembling a snail shell with 2.75 turns, the cochlea is a spiral structure, part of the membranous labyrinth. It consists of three parallel fluid-filled channels: the scala vestibuli and scala tympani which contain perilymph (similar to CSF) and the scala media or cochlear duct, which contains endo-lymph (similar in composition to intracellular fluid). Within the cochlear duct sits the long spiral set of rows of ciliated hair cells of the organ of Corti, the auditory sense receptor (see Figures 100 and 101).

The organ of Corti consists of about 35,000 hair cells which generate action potentials in the neurons of the spiral ganglion of the cochlear nerve when the hair cells are forced to vibrate by incoming sound.

Vibration proceeds through tympanic membrane, malleus, incus, and stapes in turn, is transmitted to the perilymph of the scala vestibuli, travels along the spiral of the cochlea to a point corresponding to the frequency,

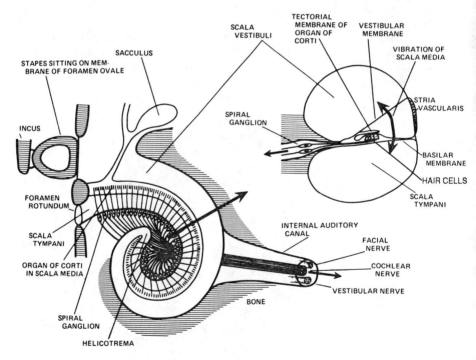

FIGURE 100. Cochlea, in plan and in cross-section. The number of turns has been abbreviated. Note that the perilymph-containing scala vestibuli and scala tympani join at the apex of the cochlea — the helicotrema. The foramen rotundum (round window) faces on the air-filled cavity of the middle ear. Scala media and vestibular membrane are often called cochlear duct and Reissner's membrane respectively.

crosses the scala media, then back along the scala tympani to the foramen rotundum (round window) whose membrane faces on the cavity of the middle ear (Figure 100). In the cochlea, the vibration takes the form of a standing wave that stimulates the hair cells of the organ of Corti maximally at one specific point along the cochlea for each frequency of incoming sound. Highest frequencies stimulate near the foramen ovale (basal cochlea), lowest frequencies at the helicotrema or apical end of cochlea.

This normal sequence is called 'air conduction.' Deafness due to lesions of external or middle ear structures is called 'conduction deafness.' (See Clinical Example 34.) Sound vibration can also arrive at the organ of Corti directly through vibration of bone, as by placing a vibrating tuning fork on the mastoid. This mechanism is called 'bone conduction.' Normally, air conduction is much more efficient than bone conduction—often abbreviated AC>BC. With nerve deafness (Clinical Example 34) both AC and BC will be diminished.

Vibration of the organ of Corti induces the cochlear microphonic, a generator potential which exactly duplicates the sound vibration. This occurs through bending of the cilia of hair cells. Tips of the cilia are embedded in the tectorial membrane, and as the organ of Corti moves upward in its vibration, the cilia are bent against the tectorial membrane, partially depolarizing the 80 mV potential between endolymph and perilymph. This upward movement occurs during the rarefaction phase of sound vibration at the eardrum. See Figures 100 and 101.

The cochlear generator potentials produced by bending of the cilia induce action potentials in the neurons of the spiral ganglion, whose axons extend medially to enter the cranial cavity via the internal auditory meatus (Figures 3 and 100).

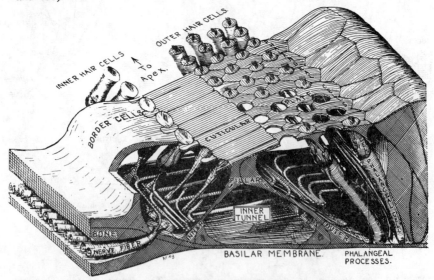

FIGURE 101. Organ of Corti. Perilymph fills the spaces (inner tunnel) below the cuticular plate, separated by tight junctions from endolymph above the plate. Tectorial membrane (not shown) lies above the hair cells to bend their cilia when the structures vibrate. (Reproduced, with permission, from Krieg: *Functional Neuroanatomy*, Brain Books, Evanston, IL.)

CENTRAL AUDITORY PATHWAYS

These axons form the cochlear nerve, and enter the brain stem at the cerebellopontine angle at the junction between medulla, pons, and cerebellum (Figures 96 and 102). At that point, the axons synapse with neurons in ventral and dorsal cochlear nuclei in the floor of the lateral recess of the fourth ventricle, partially overlying the inferior cerebellar peduncle (Figure 97).

From the ventral cochlear nucleus, second-order axons cross the midline as the trapezoid body, with synapses on neurons of the superior olivary nuclei of the same and opposite sides. At this point, the auditory projection pathway becomes bilateral. Above this level, a unilateral lesion cannot cause deafness in either ear.

From the superior olivary nucleus, axons project rostrally to the inferior colliculus via the lateral lemniscus.

From dorsal cochlear nuclei, fibers cross as the small dorsal or intermediate striae, and end on neurons of the superior olivary complex, or on other neurons such as the nucleus of the trapezoid body or of the lateral lemniscus. These connections probably have reflex functions.

CLINICAL EXAMPLE 34

A man, 53 years old, noticed that the hearing in his right ear was deteriorating. On examination, he could not hear a watch ticking when held to his right ear; the left side was normal. Conversely, a tuning fork placed on his mastoid process was heard better on the right side. Account for these findings.

Discussion

Loss of hearing in the right ear means a lesion somewhere between the right pinna and the medulla; not higher because it is unilateral. A lesion in the pathway for sound conduction from the outside to the foramen ovale causes the syndrome called conduction deafness. If the lesion is in the organ of Corti or cochlear nerve, it is called nerve deafness. The observation that he can hear in the right ear (tuning fork on mastoid) means that his right organ of Corti and nerve must be functioning, and therefore the deafness must result from problems in external or middle ear. Statistically, the most likely cause is excess wax in the ear, but in older people, otosclerosis (an arthritis of the ossicles) may cause similar effects.

Hearing via bone conduction, from the mastoid, was best on the right because of partial masking in the left ear of the tuning fork's note by extraneous noise. This is an example of lateral inhibition (see pages 70-72).

All the ascending auditory projection fibers of the lateral lemniscus relay in the inferior colliculus. Next-order fibers pass rostrally as the brachium of the inferior colliculus (inferior quadrigeminal brachium) to the medial geniculate body (MGB) of the posterior thalamus. All these structures are readily seen on the gross brain stem (Figures 96, 97, and 102).

From the MGB, axons relay laterally in the sublenticular part of the internal capsule to the lower lip of the lateral cerebral fissure (Figures 102 and

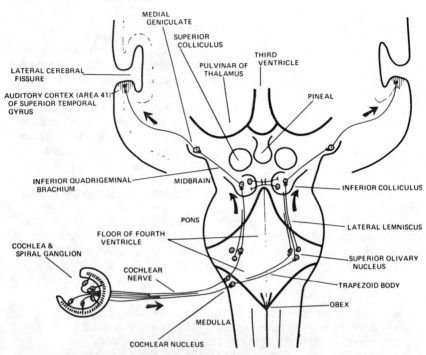

FIGURE 102. Auditory projection. Note bilaterality of projection above cochlear nuclei.

116) ending in the auditory cortex of the superior temporal gyrus (Heschl's gyrus; area 41). The projection from cochlea to cortex is tonotopically organized — each frequency corresponds to one point along the cochlea, and to one narrow strip of the auditory cortex. That is, frequency coded by location. Intensity, as in other sensory modalities, is coded by number of action potentials.

STAPEDIUS AND TENSOR TYMPANI REFLEXES

Branches of auditory fibers from cochlear nuclei synapse in the superior olivary complex of right and left sides, and relay into the adjacent reticular formation, thence into the facial (VII) and trigeminal (V) motor nuclei. Impulses from these nuclei pass peripherally to the stapedius (VII) and tensor tympani (V) muscles of the middle ear (Figure 103).

Contraction of the two muscles stretches the diarthrodial joints between the ossicles and tenses the membranes of the tympanum and of the foramen ovale, thereby decreasing energy transmission from eardrum to inner ear. This protects the inner ear from loud sounds. A person with paralysis of these muscles, or of the stapedius muscle alone (as in Bell's facial palsy) may experience the symptom of hyperacusis: sounds are perceived as uncomfortable, often louder than normal.

BLINK REFLEX

Noxious stimulation in the region of the eye causes blinking of the eyes. This has been quantitated as a standard electrophysiological test. For this test,

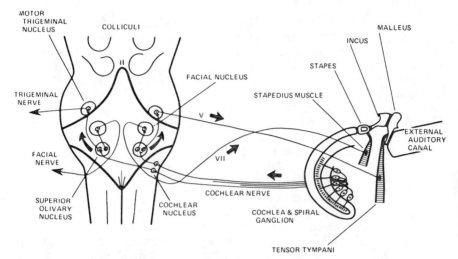

FIGURE 103. Stapedius and tensor tympani reflexes.

the supraorbital branch of the trigeminal nerve is stimulated with an electrical shock. About 10 msec later the ipsilateral eye blinks (VII facial nerve), and 30 msec after the stimulus *both* eyes blink. These long latencies indicate that the pathway from the trigeminal nucleus to the facial nucleus in the brain stem involves multiple synapses. The test is used clinically to check the intactness of this part of the brain stem (review Figures 73, 77, and 96).

LOCALIZATION OF SOUND

Sound from one side impinges on the ipsilateral and contralateral ears at slightly different times and with slightly different intensities. Incoming sounds at frequencies below 500/second appear to be localized mostly through difference in arrival time, that is, the phase of the sound wave at one ear differs from the phase at the other ear, because the distance to one ear is the width of the head farther than to the other ear. Above 1000/second, intensity becomes more important.

Bilateral interactions which mediate this localizing ability occur as low as the superior olivary nucleus (Figure 102), where each receives and integrates inputs from cochlear nuclei of both sides. Bilateral impulses interact further through the commissure of the inferior colliculus (Figure 102), to induce asymmetries in the relayed impulses. Probably commissural paths between right and left MGB, and cortical commissures such as the corpus callosum and anterior commissure are also involved. The asymmetrical impulse patterns are interpreted by cortical mechanisms as differences in azimuth.

OTHER AUDITORY REFLEXES

Reflex deviation of the eyes toward a sound occur in response to auditory impulses relayed from the inferior colliculi to the superior colliculi, thence by tectobulbar pathways as mentioned in the section on eye movements, to the extraocular muscle nuclei III, IV, and VI. The reflex may also include head turning, through tectospinal connections to cervical anterior horn cells.

Sudden convulsive contraction of many muscles in reaction to a sudden, unexpected, or loud sound, the startle reflex, probably occurs by way of similar tectospinal impulses, descending to anterior horn motoneurons the length of the spinal cord.

A small bundle of axons, the olivocochlear bundle, pass from the superior olivary complex peripherally to synapse with hair cells of the organ of Corti. Its function is not known, but it seems likely that it acts as an inhibitory sensory feedback system of some type.

VESTIBULAR RECEPTOR APPARATUS

Three semicircular canals, and a utricle and saccule comprise the five peripheral receptor organs of the vestibular system on each side (Figures 99 and 105). Being oriented in the three planes of space, the semicircular canals (superior, also called frontal or anterior; posterior, also called sagittal or inferior; and lateral, also called horizontal or external) react to rotational acceleration in any plane (see Figures 104 and 105). In an expansion of each canal, the ampulla, lies a crista, consisting of hair cells with overlying gel (cupula) extending into the endolymph of the canal. When rotational acceleration in the plane of the canal causes inertial movement of endolymph through the ampulla, bending the cilia, potentials are generated in the hair cells (Figure 106).

In the utricle and saccule, hair cells lie in two maculae, respectively horizontally and vertically oriented. Cilia of macular hair-cells are also embedded in a gel-like matrix which contains concretions of calcium carbonate (otoconia). Linear acceleration, including gravity, results in bending of the cilia by the mass of the otoconia. Thus, the semicircular canals respond primarily to rotational acceleration, the maculae of utricle and saccule to static head position

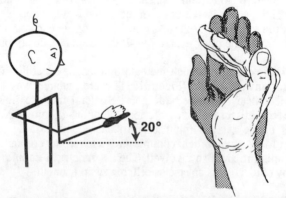

FIGURE 104. 'Handy' to demonstrate the relations of the semicircular canals in the upright head. For the canals on the left side, extend the left hand forward with palm and fingers flat, palm up, and tilted upward about 20 degrees. The plane of the palm then corresponds to the plane of the left lateral or horizontal canal. Then place the cupped right hand, fingers, and palm at right angles to each other, on the extended left hand as sketched. The plane of the right fingers then corresponds to the plane of the superior canal, and the plane of the right palm to the plane of the posterior canal.

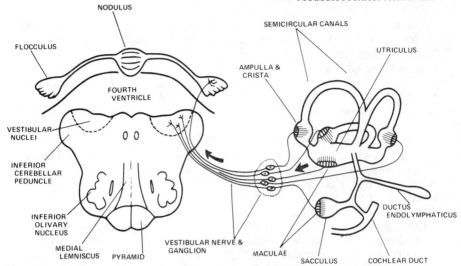

FIGURE 105. Peripheral vestibular connections. Impulses arising in the five collections of hair cells of the vestibular apparatus terminate in vestibular nuclei or in flocculonodular lobe of the cerebellum.

or rectilinear movement, i.e., linear acceleration including gravity. Examine Figures 105 and 106.

Potentials from the five hair-cell organs initiate action potentials which pass medially via axons of the bipolar neurons of the vestibular (Scarpa's) ganglion, entering the medulla at the cerebellopontine angle (Figures 96 and 105). They terminate on neurons of the four vestibular nuclei: superior, inferior (spinal), medial, and lateral (Deiter's). Other fibers bypass the nuclei to enter the flocculonodular lobe of the cerebellum.

VESTIBULAR EFFERENT CONNECTIONS

The vestibular nuclei have five types of efferent connections: first, via the MLF (Figure 98) to oculomotor nuclei III, IV, and VI; and to cranial nerve XI and anterior horn cells of the cervical cord, to adjust head and eye position in response to position and movement of the head.

The second major group of connections of vestibular nuclei are with the fastigial nuclei of the cerebellum in the roof (tectum) of the fourth ventricle. These will be discussed in the chapter on the cerebellum.

The third major connections of the vestibular system are with the reticular formation of the brain stem.

Reticular formation is the name applied to a profuse longitudinal collection of interneurons that fill the central core of the brain stem and spinal cord, with connections in many directions, and with many functions. Many reticular neurons form functional groups near cranial nerve nuclei to perform functions related to those cranial nerves.

A prominent example of this kind of relation is the vomiting center, a group of reticular neurons in the medulla near the dorsal motor nucleus of the vagus, whose parasympathetic axons carry motor impulses to the thoracic and abdominal viscera. The vomiting center organizes the impulses which, via the vagus and other nerves, induce reverse peristalsis of the gut, relaxation of sphincters, and contraction of the abdominal wall for vomiting. Connections from vestibular nuclei into the vomiting center probably account for the vomiting associated with motion sickness (sea-sickness).

Other vestibuloreticular connections may feed into the reticular activating system (RAS) to alert the individual, or into reticular centers for sleep. This latter may be a path for induction of relaxation by a rocking cradle or rocking chair.

Fourth, rostral projections through which vertigo appears as a sensory perception (dizziness) are not yet completely defined, but possibly ascend in the lateral lemniscus.

The fifth major vestibular outflow consists of the lateral vestibulospinal tract from the lateral vestibular (Deiter's) nucleus and the medial vestibulo-spinal tract from the medial vestibular nucleus. Both descend in the anterior white matter of the cord to terminate in relation to cervical motoneurons for the control of head position, particularly in response to vestibular stimulation. The lateral tract also innervates AHC to extensor muscles of the limbs for maintenance of upright posture. Vestibular or cerebellar lesions on one side will often cause the patient to hold his head in a tilted posture and to fall to that side, through abnormal impulses descending these pathways.

A memory aid: there are 5 peripheral vestibular receptors, their central axons terminate in 5 major regions, and from the vestibular nuclei there are 5 major outflows.

CLINICAL EXAMPLE 35

A man came to the clinic because of gradual loss of hearing in his right ear. As part of his examination, a caloric test was done: warm water was washed into his external auditory meatus. On the left, this caused nystagmus associated with severe vertigo. On the right, neither nystagmus nor vertigo resulted. Interpret these observations.

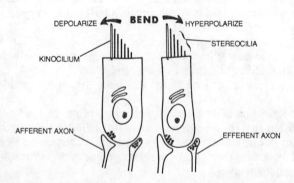

FIGURE 106. Hair cells, such as found in the cristae of the semicircular canals, the maculae of the utricle and saccule, and in the organ of Corti. Note that bending the cilia toward the kinocilium depolarizes the hair cell membrane, the other direction of bending results in hyperpolarization.

Discussion

Warmth from the water caused convection currents in the endolymph of the patient's vertical semicircular canal, with resultant vestibular impulses via MLF to the oculomotor nuclei III, IV, and VI, causing nystagmus, which is the jerky movement of the eyes by which one maintains visual fixation on moving objects. This procedure is called the 'caloric test.'

The vertigo probably was secondary to the nystagmus, though some of this sensation could be a direct vestibular effect. Absence of nystagmus on the right is abnormal, indicating damage to the peripheral organ (semicircular canal) or vestibular nerve on the right. Compare Clinical Example 37.

CLINICAL EXAMPLE 36

A 58-year-old man came in because of episodes of severe nausea and vomiting for three weeks. He had had some ringing in the right ear (tinnitus). On examination, he had a mild right nerve deafness, his right caloric response was diminished, and his right face was partially paralyzed and numb. He had a mild chronic headache. Where is the lesion?

Discussion

Ringing in the ear and vomiting suggests an eighth nerve (both vestibular and cochlear) disturbance. Deafness and decreased caloric response support this. Palsy of the right face may result from damage to the nearby facial (VII) nerve, and numbness of the right face from damage to the nearby spinal tract of the trigeminal (V) nerve. Thus, the lesion is probably in the cerebellopontine angle, where all these structures are in juxtaposition. It is most likely a tumor, judging by the patient's age and the gradual onset of symptoms.

CLINICAL EXAMPLE 37

A man brought to the hospital in coma after a CVA demonstrated a normal doll's eye phenomenon: when his head was rotated passively, his eyes remained fixated in a forward direction, i.e., they did not rotate with his head. Caloric testing with the injection of warm or cool water into the external auditory meatus caused conjugate deviation of the eyes to one side.

Discussion

Both the doll's eyes phenomenon (vestibulo-ocular reflex) and conjugate deviation of the eyes on caloric stimulation of the ears indicate that the vestibular apparatus and the brain stem mechanisms for conjugate movement are intact. In other words, the lesion causing the coma has spared his brain stem. Compare Clinical Example 35.

STUDY QUESTIONS

1. Sketch, with labels, the auditory pathway from one cochlea to the auditory cortex.
2. How is sound localized?
3. What is meant by the terms air conduction and bone conduction?
4. What is meant by nerve deafness and by conduction deafness?
5. What are the major connections of the medial longitudinal fasciculus (MLF) and their functions?
6. Define hyperacusis.
7. Discuss the importance of lateral inhibition in auditory function (compare Clinical Example 34).
8. What is nystagmus?
9. Explain the caloric test.
10. What is meant by cerebellopontine angle? Why is it important?

11 Cerebellar Mechanisms

As a convenient and useful approach to the exploration of the cerebellum, it can be divided into three major components, with anatomical and functional correlations as outlined in Table 12.

Separating paleocerebellum from neocerebellum, the primary fissure can be distinguished only on sagittal sections (Figure 107). Both grossly and histologically, the structure of cerebellar folia (Latin = leaves) are the same throughout (Figure 112). The differences in function of various parts of the cerebellum (Table 12) depend on their different connections.

The term vermis can be confusing. It refers to the worm-like appearance (Latin, vermis = worm) of the paramedian portion of the cerebellum when the lateral lobes have been removed by parasagittal cuts. It has clinical pertinence, inasmuch as lesions of the vermis are likely to result in incoordination of paraxial musculature and of the speech apparatus, so that the patient cannot maintain the upright posture (truncal ataxia), and demonstrates slurred speech. In contrast, lesions of the lateral lobes usually result in lateralized incoordination; the ipsilateral limbs are ataxic.

Ataxia is defined as incoordination of voluntary movement. Any volitional movement can be involved. Ataxia of the legs leads to wide-based gait; the patient walking with feet apart for stability. Dysmetria is the inability to move an extremity acccurately to a desired point. Overcorrection of dysmetria induces ataxic intention tremor. Ataxia of speech mechanisms causes a kind of slurred, scanning speech. Ataxia of eye movements causes nystagmus, but with irregular oscillations in contrast to the rhythmic oscillations of the eyes seen with vestibular nystagmus.

Generalized ataxia calls to mind the incoordination of motor functions observed during alcohol intoxication. Alcohol disturbs function of cerebellar mechanisms, so that the drunken individual actually demonstrates cerebellar ataxia.

TABLE 12. Subdivision of the cerebellum

Phylogenetic	Anatomical	Major Connections	Type of Function
Archicerebellum	Flocculonodular lobe and Lingula	Vestibular	Posture and eye movements
Paleocerebellum	Anterior and posterior vermis	Spinal cord	Progressive movement (walking, swimming, etc.)
Neocerebellum	Lateral lobes (corpus cerebelli)	Cerebral cortex via pons	Manipulative movement and speech

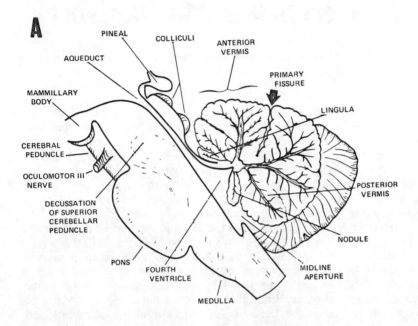

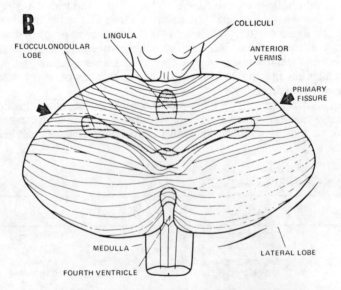

FIGURE 107. (A) midsagittal section through cerebellum and brain stem.
(B) dorsal view of the cerebellum, showing location of lingula and flocculonodular lobe (archicerebellum) as phantoms, the anterior vermis, (paleocerebellum), and the lateral lobes (neocerebellum).

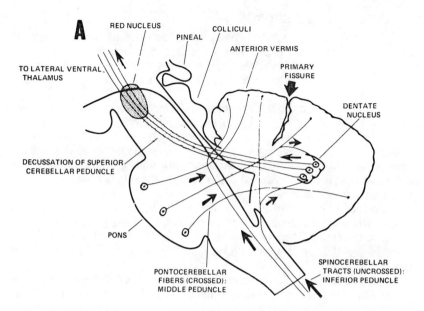

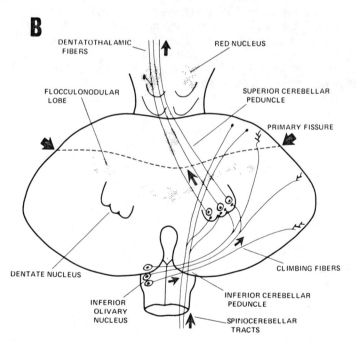

FIGURE 108. Major paleocerebellar and neocerebellar components of cerebellar peduncles. (A) Sagittal view. (B) Dorsal View.

CEREBELLAR PEDUNCLES

To introduce the cerebellar connections, first consider the three pairs of peduncles through which these connections pass in or out; inferior cerebellar peduncles (restiform body); middle cerebellar peduncles (brachium pontis); and superior cerebellar peduncles (brachium conjunctivum), see Figures 74-78, and 108).

About 40 percent of the fibers of the **inferior cerebellar peduncle** come from the ipsilateral leg with relay in the nucleus dorsalis of the spinal cord (Figure 110), or from the ipsilateral arm with relay in the lateral (external) cuneate nucleus just lateral to the cuneate nucleus in the medulla. This input is uncrossed. Most of these fibers, concerned with limb movements, go to the anterior vermis (Figures 108A and 110) rostral to the primary fissure, some go to the posterior vermis.

Another 40 percent of the fibers come from the opposite inferior olivary nucleus, which relays rostral as well as spinal cord inputs (Figures 108B and 111). The remaining fibers of the inferior peduncle are vestibular (archicerebellar, Figure 109) or connect with reticular formation of medulla and lower pons.

The **middle cerebellar peduncle** consists mostly of fibers from the pontine nuclei of the opposite side. Pontine neurons receive impulses from frontal and parietotemporal cortex including a considerable contribution from the motor cortex, and from brain stem nuclei, to coordinate delicate motor activities such as the use of fingers and speech musculature (Figures 108A and 111). The middle cerebellar peduncle is the direct lateral extension of the pons (Figures 4, 96, 108, and 111).

Most of the rostral outflow from the cerebellum exits via **superior cerebellar peduncles.** The fibers arise as axons from neurons of the roof nuclei of the cerebellum (dentate, interpositus, and fastigial nuclei) project rostrally

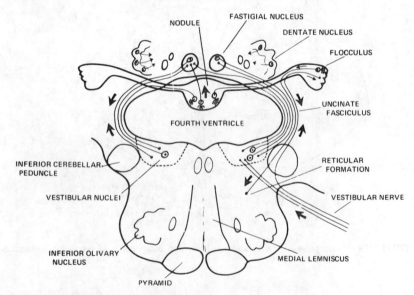

FIGURE 109. Archicerebellar connections

and ventrally into the midbrain to decussate under the inferior colliculus (Figures 78, 108, and 111). Collaterals of some of the fibers synapse with neurons in the red nucleus, from which arises the rubrospinal tract. The fibers continue to the thalamus, synapsing on neurons of the lateral ventral nucleus, to relay via the internal capsule to the motor cortex, areas 4 and 6.

Some of the spinocerebellar fibers diverge from the main dorsal spino-cerebellar tract which enters the inferior peduncle, to enter alongside the superior peduncle as the ventral spinocerebellar tract. These mostly arise from neurons in the posterior horns relaying Ib impulses from Golgi tendon organs. The ventral spinocerebellar tract is believed to carry 'efference copy' or 'corollary discharge,' by which is meant an internally directed system whose purpose is to 'report to the CNS' neural events taking place in the spinal cord.

ARCHICEREBELLUM

As suggested by Table 12, the archicerebellum (ancient cerebellum) is an evolutionary growth of the vestibular system. Some vestibular fibers go directly to the cerebellar cortex of the flocculonodular lobe and lingula, but most relay through the vestibular nuclei (Figures 105 and 109), with connections to and from fastigial nuclei of both sides.

Archicerebellar cortex acts through fastigial and vestibular nuclei to anterior horn cells of the spinal cord via vestibulospinal tracts, to oculomotor nuclei via MLF (see Figures 98 and 109), or into the reticular formation for a number of different connections.

PALEOCEREBELLUM

Incoming paleocerebellar (old cerebellar) action potentials originate from skin, joints, and primary (annulospiral) endings of the neuromuscular spindles, to enter the cord with dorsal roots. From the leg, they synapse in the nucleus dorsalis (Clarke) of the posterior horn, and ascend as the ipsilateral dorsal spinocerebellar tract on the lateral surface of the cord just ventral to the dorsal roots. From the arm, fibers ascend to synapse in the lateral cuneate nucleus in the medulla. Both relays enter the cerebellum via the ipsilateral inferior cerebellar peduncle to terminate as mossy fibers in the granule cell layer of the anterior vermis, with collaterals to roof nuclei, mostly dentate (Figures 110 and 111).

These inputs are topographically organized (Figure 115). After stimulating the neurons of the dentate nucleus, the mossy fibers stimulate granule cells of the cerebellar cortex, which in turn stimulate Purkinje cells. From the Purkinje cells then arise patterned sequences of inhibitory impulses back to the dentate nucleus, modifying its rostral outflow to the contralateral red nucleus, LV thalamus, and motor cortex. Through these connections, the cerebellum exerts a major influence on the pyramidal tract, and on both alpha and gamma anterior horn cells.

The rubrospinal tract lies just ventral to the pyramidal tract in the spinal cord, and synapses on anterior horn motoneurons. This tract is of great importance in the cat, and in humans is believed to mediate gross limb movement, in contrast to the delicate manipulative movements mediated by the pyramidal tract. Review Figures 8 and 54.

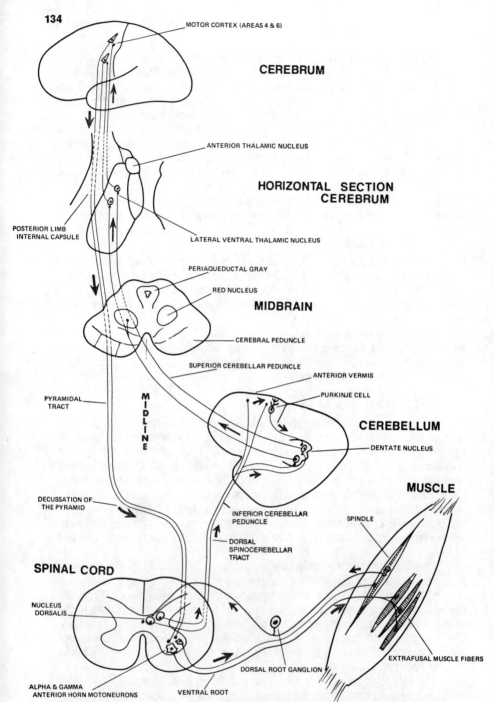

FIGURE 110. Major paleocerebellar connections. Note that cerebellar connections are on the same side as the muscle and spinal cord connections, and that midbrain, thalamic, and cortical connections are contralateral. In addition to the afferents from spindles as pictured, there are numerous inputs to the nucleus dorsalis from skin and joint receptors.

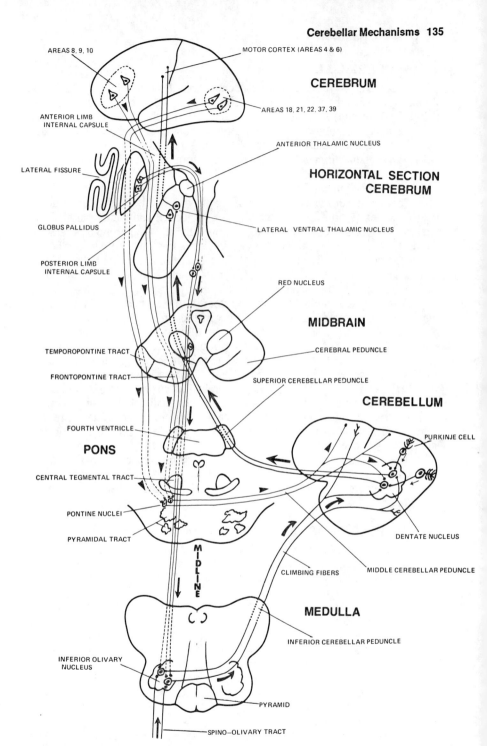

FIGURE 111. Major neocerebellar connections.

NEOCEREBELLUM

Neocerebellar (new cerebellar) connections (Figure 111), appeared in phylogeny at the time of elaboration of the cerebral cortex (neocortex) of mammals. It reaches its largest size in primates with their manipulative abilities. The neocerebellum can appropriately be thought of as the motor coordinator for hands and mouth; for manipulation and speech.

Neocerebellar inputs fall into two major groups, fibers from the pontine nuclei (pontocerebellar mossy fibers) and fibers from the inferior olivary nuclei (olivocerebellar climbing fibers).

Pontine nuclei receive synaptic inputs from frontal and parietotemporal areas of cortex (Figure 111), descending in the medial and lateral parts of the cerebral peduncles as corticopontine (frontopontine and temporopontine) tracts. Axons from pontine nuclei cross the midline to form the middle cerebellar peduncle, ascend into the lateral lobes of the cerebellum, sending collaterals to dentate nuclei, then, as mossy fibers, synapse with granule cells and Golgi cells in glomeruli of the granular layer.

A large rostral input arrives at the inferior olivary nucleus in the central tegmental tract, from red nucleus and other rostral structures. It also receives a significant input from spinal cord, the spino-olivary tract, which runs on the ventrolateral surface of the cord. The inferior olivary nucleus may be thought of as a center for interaction between rostral brain stem influences and spinal cord influences concerned with motor coordination. Fibers leaving the inferior olivary nucleus cross the midline, enter the cerebellum as part of the inferior cerebellar peduncle, send collaterals to dentate nuclei, and end in a profusion of synapses on the elaborate dendritic tree of Purkinje cells. These are the climbing fibers: one olivary neuron sends one climbing fiber which probably stimulates only one Purkinje cell.

Lesions of the corticopontine system may cause cerebellar ataxia. Frontal lobe lesions also occasionally do so. Lesions of the central tegmental tract (see Figure 77) cause a peculiar movement disorder of the throat called palatal myoclonus.

HISTOLOGY OF THE CEREBELLUM

As commented earlier, all folia consist of the same cellular components. So far as is known, all function the same way. Even more interestingly, the basic cellular pattern shows only relatively minor differences in vastly different members of the vertebrate phylum.

Figures 112 and 113 and Table 13 should be studied together for the following discussion.

One climbing fiber stimulates roof nuclei (dentate, interpositus, or fastigial) then stimulates one Purkinje cell through its hundreds of synapses scattered all over the massive Purkinje cell dendritic tree. Occasional climbing fibers also stimulate Golgi cells and probably basket and stellate cells.

Each mossy fiber stimulates roof nuclei, then excites a number of glomeruli in the granule cell layer of several adjacent folia, specifically activating granule cell and Golgi cell dendrites within the glomerulus.

Activated granule cell axons extend toward the surface as parallel fibers, running the length of a folium for 3-5 mm, and exciting Purkinje cell dendrites as well as basket and stellate cells. The elaborate espalier-like Purkinje cell

TABLE 13. Cerebellar cortex; cell types and interactions

Cell types	Interactions
Climbing fiber	Excites roof nuclei, Purkinje cell, Golgi cell
Mossy fiber	Excites roof nuclei, granule cells, Golgi cells
Granule cell (parallel fiber)	Excites Purkinje cells, basket cells, stellate cells, Golgi cells
Golgi cell	Inhibits granule cells (glomeruli)
Basket cell	Inhibits Purkinje cells (basal)
Stellate cell	Inhibits Purkinje cells (dendritic)
Purkinje cell	Inhibits Golgi cells, roof nuclei, lateral vestibular nuclei, and other Purkinje cells

dendritic tree extends at right angles to the long axis of the folium, and therefore at right angles to parallel fibers. As many as 100,000 parallel fibers synapse with dendritic spines on the elaborate dendritic tree of the Purkinje cell.

Golgi cells, excited by climbing fibers, by mossy fibers, and by parallel fibers, send inhibitory axons into the glomerulus to inhibit granule cells, then they in turn are inhibited by Purkinje cell axon collaterals.

Basket cells, excited slightly later, strongly inhibit Purkinje cells through a basket-like array of axon terminals arranged around the Purkinje cell axon hillock. Stellate cells also inhibit Purkinje cell activity, but at the dendritic end.

As a result of all these interactions, incoming climbing fiber and mossy fiber excitatory volleys cause an outgoing inhibitory volley from Purkinje cells, then immediately turns off the whole mechanism in preparation for the next volley, a few milliseconds later. Evidently, the cerebellar cortex acts as a modulating computer, adjusting the excitatory output of the roof nuclei or of the lateral vestibular nucleus or reticular formation (Figure 114). The secondary importance of the cerebellar cortex is emphasized by the clinical observation that isolated damage to the cortex usually causes only mild ataxia, while lesions damaging roof nuclei invariably cause very severe and usually permanent ataxia.

SOMATOTOPIC REPRESENTATION OF CEREBELLAR CORTEX

Both paleocerebellar and neocerebellar cortices relate point-to-point with regions of the body on the same side (Figure 115). This is grossly observed in the projection from ipsilateral leg via dorsal spinocerebellar tract, and from ipsilateral arm via cuneocerebellar tract, from lateral cuneate nucleus. These relationships account for localization of ataxia from cerebellar lesions. Lateral lesions cause ataxia of ipsilateral arm, leg, or both. Midline (vermis) lesions lead to ataxia of paraxial musculature, disturbing upright posture, or to ataxia of speech (Clinical Examples 38 and 39).

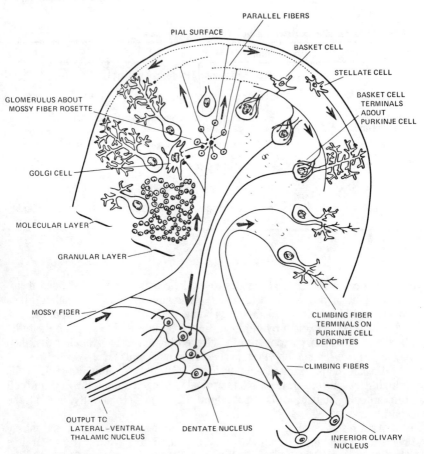

FIGURE 112. Histology of a cerebellar folium. Section at right angles to long axis of the folium. The parallel fiber axons of granular cells are indicated in dashed lines because they actually run parallel to the long axis of the folium (at right angles to the plane of the diagram).

CEREBELLAR COORDINATION OF MOVEMENT

Cerebellar outflows modulate both alpha and gamma motoneuron function through several paths. Probably the most important is the rostral projection via dentatothalamic route to the motor cortex, directly affecting pyramidal function. Lesions in this outflow manifest the most severe ataxia.

From pontine reticular formation, numerous mossy fibers enter the cerebellum. Other reticular nuclei receive cerebellar outputs. Some of these project downstream as reticulospinal tracts, acting again on both alpha and gamma motoneurons. The general effect on gamma motoneurons is excitatory—cerebellar lesions decrease this excitation, causing muscular hypotonus, meaning decreased maintenance of reflex postural tension.

Vestibulocerebellar impulses descend the lateral vestibulospinal tract for contraction of extensor muscles to maintain upright posture. Patients with

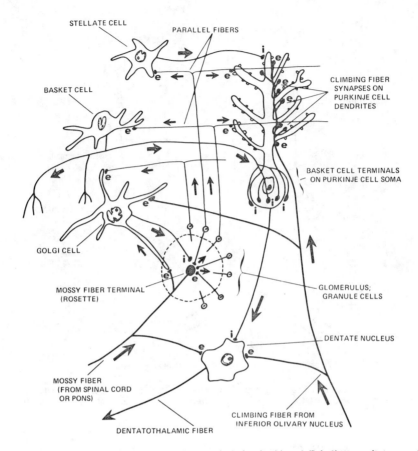

FIGURE 113. Summary of major cerebellar cortical circuits (e) and (i) indicate excitatory and inhibitory synapses, respectively. (Correlate with Figure 112.)

lesions in the vestibulocerebellar system on one side often tilt the head to that side, and may fall to that side. This has been described as loss of extensor tone.

Rubrospinal connections relay from cerebellum, but may be of minor importance in humans. Because of the overlap between rubrospinal and lateral corticospinal tracts in the human spinal cord, it has been impossible to differentiate the contributions of the two tracts with certainty (Figures 8 and 54).

Finally, the loop of interconnections between cerebral cortex and cerebellar cortex, the cortico-ponto-cerebello-dentato-thalamo-cortical circuit, is felt by many to be the system through which repeated volitional movements become habitual or 'learned.' By this hypothesis, a complex movement, such as writing one's name, at first depends entirely on volitional cortical outputs. With many repetitions, circuits develop which may then be triggered volitionally to carry out the desired movement automatically.

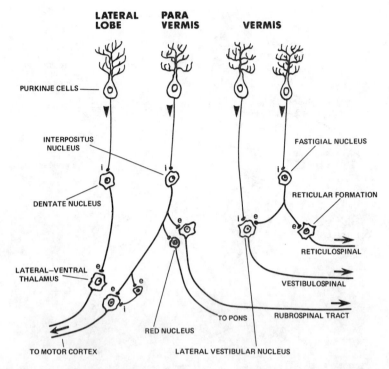

FIGURE 114. Summary of major projections from Purkinje cells, the cerebellar cortical outflow pathways. Excitatory synapses are indicated by (e) and inhibitory synapses by (i).

GLOMERULUS

As a neuroanatomical and neurophysiological concept, the glomerulus has assumed great importance. For example, glomeruli of the granule cell layer of the cerebellar cortex consist of three major components: mossy fiber excitatory synapses, granule cell and Golgi cell dendrites, and Golgi cell inhibitory axon terminals. In other words, this structure, some distance from nerve cell bodies, has all the synaptic functional characteristics of nerve cell bodies, making possible excitation, inhibition, and summation. Because the number of glomeruli may be many times the number of cell bodies, this multiplies the available functioning units many-fold.

CLINICAL EXAMPLE 38

A man, 43 years old, began to stumble frequently, and fell several times. His problem culminated when he was arrested for drunkenness, even though he had not been drinking or taking any drug.
On examination, he was upset, and spoke in a slurred, somewhat explosive manner. His strength was good, but when asked to do the finger-to-nose test, he missed his nose, and developed a

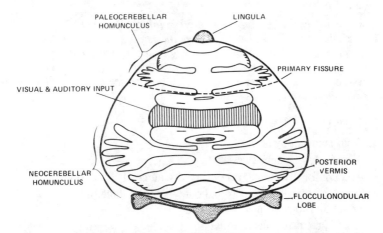

FIGURE 115. Topographic localization in the cerebellar cortex, modified from Snider for the monkey. Humans probably have similar patterns. Note the two homunculi, and the separate region for auditory and visual projection. Vestibular inputs go to the archicerebellum = flocculonodular lobe and lingula.

severe irregular hand tremor as his finger approached his nose. Pronation-supination of both hands was slow and uncoordinated (dysdiadochokinesia). He walked unsteadily, swaying irregularly and planting his feet wide apart. On lateral gaze, his eyes jerked irregularly.

Discussion

All of the findings described: slurred, explosive speech, intention tremor on finger-to-nose testing, dysmetria ('he missed his nose'), dysdiadochokinesia, unsteady wide-based gait, and irregular nystagmus on lateral gaze, characterize cerebellar ataxia. From the protocol, the ataxia appears to be generalized, not lateralized or focal. Probably the entire cerebellum is damaged.

This sort of cerebellar disease may result from toxic reactions to chemicals or drugs, to spontaneous cerebellar degeneration, or to inherited cerebellar disease. Under the microscope, this gentleman's cerebellum would probably show diffuse loss of Purkinje cells and/or granule cells.

CLINICAL EXAMPLE 39

Following an auto accident, a 17-year-old girl was comatose for a week, then gradually recovered. After several months, her right arm, and to some extent right leg demonstrated dysmetria, intention tremor, and incoordination of rapid alternating movements. Speech was a bit slow. All other neurological testing gave normal results.

Discussion

Long-lasting coma indicates severe brain injury. The neuro-logical abnormalities in her right arm and leg are attributable to right-sided cerebellar damage, involving arm area more than leg area. Slowness of speech may also be a cerebellar sign, though with a severe brain injury, damage to the cerebral cortex may cause the slowed speech.

STUDY QUESTIONS

1. What is meant by ataxia?
2. What is dysdiadochokinesia?
3. Account for the nystagmus observed with cerebellar lesions.
4. Sketch and label the inputs and outputs of the three functional divisions of the cerebellum.
5. What is the cerebellar vermis?
6. Outline the connections through which the cerebellum acts ipsilaterally on motor function.
7. From which peripheral end-organs do cerebellar inputs originate?
8. Sketch the gross morphology of the cerebellum with labels.
9. Outline, on a sketch of the cerebellar cortex, the somatotopic projections (homunculi).
10. List the five neuronal cell types in cerebellar cortex.
11. What are mossy and climbing fibers?
12. Describe the connections and effects of each of the neuronal cell types in cerebellar cortex.
13. Describe the function of the cerebellar computer at a cellular level.

12 Cerebral Cortex

In the hierarchy of the central nervous system, the cerebral cortex is considered highest, assuming the supreme importance of symbolic functions such as speech, mathematical manipulation, artistic activities, and intellection. The cerebral cortex mediates these functions; it is the most human part of the brain.

Right and left cerebral hemispheres fill the entire cranial cavity above the tentorium, the supratentorial compartment (Figure 31). Each hemisphere consists of a superficial layer of neurons 3-5 mm thick, the cerebral cortex, a tremendous mass of underlying myelinated axons, the white matter (connections to, from, and between cortical areas), and large subcortical nuclei; thalamus, hypothalamus, subthalamus, and basal ganglia.

GROSS MORPHOLOGY OF THE CEREBRUM

Total area of cortex approximates 2000 square centimeters, and it is folded into numerous ridges or convolutions, the gyri, which are separated by infolded crevasses, sulci and fissures. The foldings result from overgrowth of the cerebral cortex relative to the bony cranium. With a few important exceptions, gyri and sulci are inconstant. Figures 1, 2, 116, and 117 outline the boundaries of the major cortical subdivisions, the lobes, and many of the gyri and sulci.

FRONTAL LOBE

Cortex behind the forehead makes up the frontal lobe, bounded below by the lateral fissure (Sylvius) and behind by the central sulcus (Rolando). The precentral gyrus, on the anterior lip of the central sulcus, is already familiar as the primary motor cortex, Brodmann's area 4 (Figures 50 and 116). Area 6, premotor cortex, just in front of area 4, also gives rise to pyramidal tract fibers. Area 8, still more rostral, controls adversive conjugate deviation of the eyes (Figure 116). All three of these areas extend over the superior edge of the hemisphere into the midline longitudinal fissure (Figure 117).

Broca's area 44, immediately in front of the motor areas for face (lower ends of areas 4 and 6, next to the lateral fissure), is historically important as the first cortical region whose associational function was defined. More than 100 years ago, Broca pointed out that lesions here cause the speech disturbance called expressive aphasia.

Orbital gyri, on the undersurfaces of the frontal lobe, lie directly on the orbital bone, and with the parolfactory cortex inferior to the genu of the corpus callosum, are part of the limbic system. The subcallosal gyrus lies immediately below the genu. Orbital cortex may be important in cortical activation via the reticular activating system, as will be discussed later.

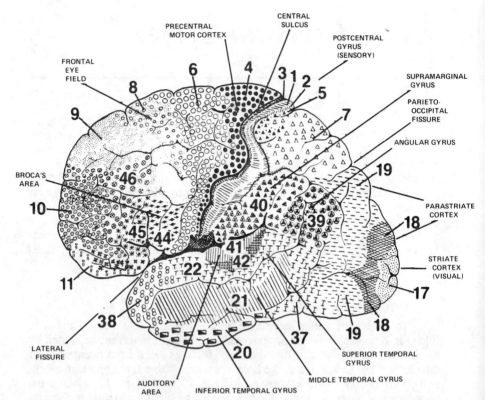

FIGURE 116. Major cytoarchitectonic areas of the cortex, convex (lateral) surface. After Brodmann. (Correlate with Figure 1.)

The frontopontine tract, which relays via pons to cerebellar cortex, arises from area 8 and areas 9 and 10 of the frontal pole.

Most of the frontal cortex appears to mediate higher level functions, providing a basis for social interactions and recognition of cause and effect relations. Fibers interconnecting frontal cortex and thalamus are severed in the operation of frontal lobotomy or leucotomy.

PARIETAL LOBE

From the central sulcus, the parietal lobe extends backward to the parieto-occipital fissure on the medial surface. On the lateral surface, no gross landmarks separate it from occipital and posterior temporal lobes. Its inferior border is a backward continuation of the lateral fissure.

Motor and sensory cortex for the opposite leg and genital region form the paracentral lobule, including cortex both on frontal lobe and parietal lobe sides of the central sulcus on the medial surface of the hemisphere (Figure 117). It lies only a few millimeters from the paracentral lobule of the opposite hemisphere, separated only by meninges including the falx, and CSF. Expanding tumors here can damage both sides, to cause paralysis and sensory loss in both legs. Such parasagittal lesions may be confused with spinal cord lesions.

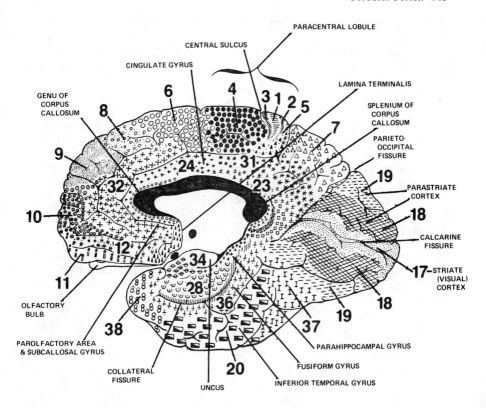

FIGURE 117. Major cytoarchitectonic areas of the cortex, medial surface. After Brodmann. (Correlate with Figures 2, 4, and 118.)

Areas 3-1-2 run the length of the postcentral gyrus, and receive the cortical projection of somatic sensation from the opposite side of the body, in inverted orientation, see Figures 62 and 63.

Areas 40 and 39, the supramarginal and angular gyri, apparently interpret incoming sensory stimuli. Lesions usually cause agnosias: aphasias, apraxia, atopognosia, etc. They lie just behind the sensory area for face, and between it and the visual cortex of the occipital lobe. Areas 40, 39, and part of 22 in the temporal lobe constitute Wernicke's area for speech.

OCCIPITAL LOBE

Visual functions occupy the entire occipital lobe. Striate cortex (area 17, visual cortex, calcarine cortex) makes up the upper and lower lips of the calcarine fissure. From upper retina, optic impulses project to the upper lip; from lower retina, to the lower lip of the fissure, mapping the contralateral visual hemi-fields of both eyes (Figure 90).

Parastriate cortex, Brodmann's areas 18 and 19, receive secondary projections from the primary visual cortex, area 17. The projection into area 18 is oriented as in area 17, and is inverted in area 19. These areas mediate accommodation reflexes and eye movements, and take part in interpretation of visual inputs (Figures 93 and 95).

As part of the oculomotor control system, area 18 is connected with area 8, frontal eye field, by a large bundle of fibers, the superior longitudinal fasciculus (Figures 95 and 121).

TEMPORAL LOBE

The temporal lobe lies below the lateral fissure and to the side of the brain stem, which it partially surrounds laterally.

Area 41, the auditory projection cortex, lies horizontally inside the lateral fissure on the upper surface of the superior temporal gyrus. It cannot be seen without opening the fissure. Adjacent para-auditory cortex, areas 42 and 22, of superior and middle temporal gyri, lie on the lateral surface. Lesions in these areas, on the left side of the brain, often cause auditory agnosia — the inability to understand speech even with relatively normal hearing acuity.

At the anterior end of the parahippocampal gyrus, the mesial temporal cortex lying next to the brain stem, is found the uncus, which receives projection fibers for the sense of smell from the olfactory bulb on the same side. It consists mostly of cortex associated with the limbic system (Figures 4, 80, 117, 118, and 124).

Grossly, the gyri of the temporal lobe can be pictured as five parallel fingers extending forward from the occipital region toward the temporal pole (Figure 118).

In the depths of the temporal lobe on the floor of the temporal horn of the lateral ventricle (Figure 118) lies the hippocampus, an important component of the limbic system. The name derives from a fancied resemblance of its cross-section to the sea horse. The hippocampus is three-layered archicortex (ancient cortex) and appears important in recent memory, memory retained for 5-10 minutes. The amygdala or amygdaloid nuclear complex, another major component of the limbic system, lies rostral to the hippocampus, just above the tip of the temporal horn, and immediately deep to the uncus. It has many connections with all these structures.

The cingulate gyrus, extending from frontal into parietal lobe on the medial surface, just above the corpus callosum, is also limbic (Figures 117 and 121) with connections into the hippocampus. Thus the temporal lobe includes functional areas for hearing, vision, olfaction, and limbic system.

INSULA

Spreading the lips of the lateral fissure exposed the insula, hidden by overlying flaps (opercula, Latin = gills) of frontal cortex, parietal cortex, and temporal cortex. Figure 118 shows this relation.

Insular cortex appears to be motor and sensory for visceral structures. Electrical stimulation of the region at surgery has been observed to cause borborygmus (stomach rumbling = increased peristaltic activity). The common epigastric sensation premonitory to many epileptic seizures may result from involvement of insular cortex in the seizure discharge.

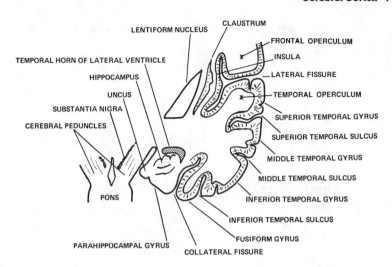

FIGURE 118. Coronal section through one temporal lobe at the level of the uncus. Note that the hippocampus is infolded, forming part of the floor of the temporal horn of the lateral ventricle.

HISTOLOGY OF THE NEOCORTEX

Neocortex or neopallium is ordinarily described as being made up of six layers or laminae. In contrast, the limbic archicortex has three layers. Neocortical layering is somewhat arbitrary, and the pattern varies from region to region. Some samples are sketched in Figure 119.

A variety of ways of categorizing cortical regions has been devised, depending on cellular organization or fiber content. In the early 1900s, some workers defined up to 200 different types of cortex. Insamuch as function appears only roughly correlated with this aspect of cortical organization, nowadays this multiplicity does not seem useful. Probably as few as three to five histologically defined types of cortex suffice. Specifically motor cortex is often called agranular (Figure 119) because of its relatively small number of granule cells. Sensory projection areas are called granular or koniocortex because of the predominance of these small neurons.

Laminar fiber patterns are also of interest, but are rarely used in classification, with the exception of the stria of Gennari in layer IV of visual cortex. See Table 14.

By using special cell stains, it can be shown that neurons of the cortex synapse with each other in a bewildering variety of ways. Figure 120 suggests some interconnections within a small cortical region.

Connections as depicted in Figure 120 number 10,000 to 100,000 per individual cortical neuron. Calculating from the cortical population, averaging about 50,000 neurons per square millimeter of cortical surface, the number of synaptic interconnections is seen to be tremendous. Direct counting from electron micrographs indicate about 10^9 (one billion) synapses per cubic millimeter of cortex. Multiplied by the total cortical volume of about 500,000 cubic millimeters, leads to about 10^{15} (one quadrillion = one million billion) synaptic interconnections in the human neocortex alone!

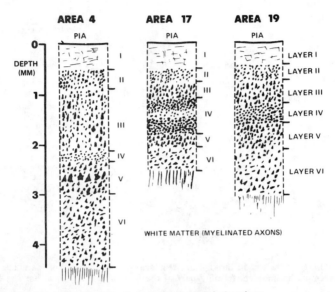

FIGURE 119. Cellular lamination of representative cortical regions.

Area 4 — Motor cortex or agranular cortex contains few granule cells in layer IV. Note the giant pyramidal cells of Betz in layer V.

Area 17 — Visual sensory area is granular cortex or koniocortex. Very few pyramidal cells, and many granule cells in layer IV.

Area 19 — Association cortex is intermediate between motor and sensory cortex.

TABLE 14. Functional connections of neocortical layers

Layer	
I	**Molecular layer.** Contains terminal dendrites and many axons of cortical neurons, as an elaborate neuropil in which numerous interconnections occur.
II	**Outer granular layer.** Receives major inputs from other cortical regions. Receptor cortex characteristically has many granule cells. (Also called stellate cells.)
III	**Outer pyramidal layer.** Contains somewhat larger pyramidal-shaped neurons whose axons go to other cortical regions.
IV	**Inner granular layer.** Many granule cells receiving major thalamic inputs, as well as inputs from other subcortical nuclei. In this layer is the prominent band of myelinated fibers called the stria of Gennari of the calcarine cortex.
V	**Inner pyramidal layer or ganglion layer.** Contains many large pyramidal cells, including the giant cells of Betz, which occur almost entirely in the motor cortex, area 4. These large cells' axons extend to distant subcortical neurons, e.g., to spinal cord motoneurons via the pyramidal tract.
VI	**Multiform layer.** Neurons of various sizes and shapes, evidently mostly mediating intercortical or intracortical connections, and connection to the same region of the thalamus from which the inputs to Layer IV originate.

Exactly what these multitudinous synapses accomplish and how they operate remains unknown in detail. We can, however, safely assume that they mediate the almost infinite variety of mental and other human functions that we perform so readily.

RADIAL OR COLUMNAR ORGANIZATION OF NEOCORTEX

Bundles of fibers enter the cortex and depart in radial fashion — at right angles to the pial surface. This, together with the point-to-point mapping of visual and other sensory and motor regions, suggests that columns of cortical neurons may be organized relative to these points. About 20 years ago, Hubel and Wiesel demonstrated in the cat's visual cortex that such organization does indeed obtain.

Using microelectrodes to record from single neurons, they showed that each neuron in a column of cells about 1 mm across responds to visual events occurring at one point in the visual field. Each 1-mm column is made up of an 0.5-mm column from each eye, the ocular dominance columns (see Figure 87). These larger columns are made up of single-neuron columns of cells extending through the cortex, all of which respond to edges or bars of light with the same geometric orientation. Adjacent single-neuron columns respond to slightly different orientations, and so on across the 0.5-mm column to complete a full 180 degree change in orientation. Thus, each 0.5-mm ocular dominance column contains sets of neurons capable of responding to linear visual stimuli of all possible orientations. Individual cells within the single-cell column respond to specific kinds of visual event: movement, dark edge, light edge, linear stimuli of fixed length, color, etc., but always with the same visual orientation.

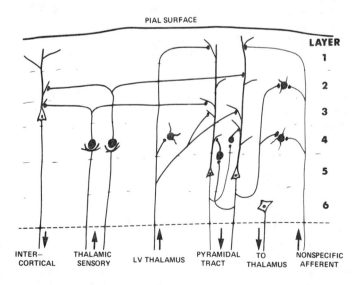

FIGURE 120. Some major neocortical connections, greatly simplified. Solid black neurons represent the very numerous intrinsic cortical neurons, which have no extracortical connections.

These ocular dominance columns, and analogous columns in other sensory or motor areas probably mediate the most direct intracortical cross-talk. Possible examples: binocular vision in the visual cortex, recognition that one point touched is adjacent to another in the somatosensory area.

SECONDARY MOTOR AND SENSORY AREAS

Most, if not all, motor and sensory functions are multiply-represented in the neocortex. Secondary motor and sensory areas maintain point-to-point relations with the external world. The secondary homunculi derived from these relationships tend to be more distorted than the primary sensory or motor areas, they occupy less space, and often project bilaterally to some degree. The secondary motor area lies at the inferior end of the postcentral gyrus, overlapping the lower end of the somatosensory cortex; the supplementary motor area lies on the medial surface of the hemisphere just in front of the paracentral lobule.

CLINICAL EXAMPLE 40

A gentleman suffered a stroke, followed by several days of coma. As he recovered, he showed left-sided weakness, and it was noted that when a pencil or similar object was placed in his left palm, his hand closed on it automatically. Discuss this phenomenon.

Discussion

Automatic grasping of this type is called the 'grasp reflex.' It is an example of an infantile reflex; the baby's reflex holding on to mother to keep from falling. The reflex normally disappears with maturity, apparently inhibited by innervations from the supplementary motor area, in a manner analogous to the inhibition of the withdrawal plantar reflex (Babinski reflex) by the primary motor cortex.

In this patient, the grasp reflex probably resulted from damage to the supplementary motor area by the vascular lesion of the frontal lobe.

Ten different areas have been demonstrated to relate to the primary visual inputs, eight cortical projections exist for hearing. At least three such areas have been defined for every motor and sensory area, and many neurons in association areas respond specifically to more than one sensory input. A reasonable deduction from these data is that nearly every cortical region receives indirect inputs from every sensory system, and sends indirect impulses to every motor region.

This idea of cortical pluripotency will be further explored in the later section on hologram analogy.

INTER- AND INTRACORTICAL FIBER PATHS

Figure 120 depicts intracortical connections within a given cortical area. Somewhat longer fiber bundles connect adjacent cortical regions. These U fibers loop down into the white matter, then immediately back into the cortex a few millimeters away (Figure 121). U fibers may remain undamaged in diseased brains where the deep white matter has degenerated because of vascular or other lesions (see Figure 22).

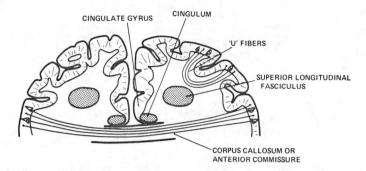

FIGURE 121. Coronal section showing three types of intercortical fiber connections: local U fibers, symmetrical side-to-side fibers via the corpus callosum, and two long anterior to posterior bundles. See also Figures 95, 123, 124, 128, and 129.

Two important sets of U fibers are the massive interconnections across the central sulcus between motor and sensory cortex in both directions, and the organized connections between striate and parastriate cortices, areas 17, 18, and 19.

Longer fiber pathways connect related cortical areas at greater distances. For instance, the frontal eye field (area 8) and parastriate cortex of the occipital lobe (area 18), both of which are concerned with eye movements, are connected by the massive bundle of intracortical fibers called the superior longitudinal fasciculus (Figures 95 and 121). A massive bundle connects Broca's area for motor speech, area 44, with Wernicke's sensory areas for speech, areas 40, 39, 22, 42. The inferior longitudinal fasciculus connects anterior temporal cortex with posterior temporal and occipital cortex. The uncinate fasciculus connects frontal and temporal cortex. Curving within the cingulate gyrus, the cingulum connects with limbic structures such as the hippocampus deep in the temporal lobe (Figures 121 and 142). Most impressive of all, the corpus callosum interconnects right and left hemispheres (Figures 121 and 123).

CEREBRAL COMMISSURES

The corpus callosum is the largest single fiber bundle in the entire nervous system Its fibers connect symmetrical cortical areas of right and left hemispheres (Figures 121 and 123). Parts of specific motor and sensory areas, areas 17, 4, 3-1-2, 41, are not so connected; but the adjacent areas, 6, 8, 42, etc. are massively represented. This emphasis on association cortex makes sense in light of the known function of the corpus callosum, which is the transfer of learned information from one side to the other. Epileptic seizures also may spread via the same path from one side to the other, so callosotomy has occasionally been used in treatment of intractable spells.

Homologous with the corpus callosum, the anterior commissure connects middle temporal gyri of the two sides (Figure 124). It also includes limbic system connections between amygdaloid nuclei and olfactory bulbs of the two sides, as well as fibers from the hippocampus via the fornix to the opposite hypothalamus and septum.

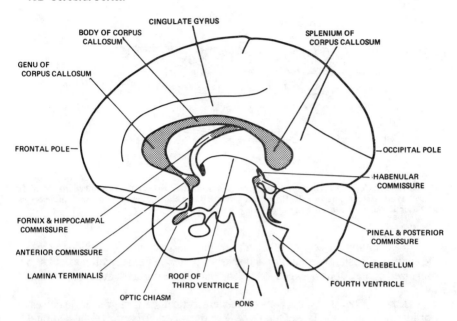

FIGURE 122. Medial view of right cerebral hemisphere showing the telencephalic commissures: corpus callosum, anterior commissure, and hippocampal commissure; and the diencephalic commissures: optic chiasm, habenular commissure, and posterior commissure.

Possibly concerned with recent memory, the hippocampal commissure connects one hippocampus with the other. These structures are also limbic (Figure 124). The habenular commissure connects right and left habenular nuclei, limbic structures located at the caudal end of the roof of the third ventricle (Figure 122).

Running with the optic chiasm are two small commissures, Gudden's and Meynert's, of uncertain significance.

As a frequently cited neuroanatomical landmark, the posterior commissure marks the caudal end of the third ventricle. It carries fibers for the pupillary light reflex, and for the medial longitudinal fasciculus (Figures 92, 95, and 122).

HEMISPHERIC INDEPENDENCE — THE SPLIT BRAIN

As mentioned, the corpus callosum and other commissures may be sectioned to prevent the spread of epileptic seizures across the midline. Psychological examination of such split-brain patients reveals unexpected independence of function of the two hemispheres. Each hemisphere, separately, appears to have the ability to remember, to respond emotionally, and to function in motor, sensory, and intellectual spheres. Each half-brain receives, recalls, interprets, and responds to inputs independently of the other.

This independence can be demonstrated by asking such a patient to close his eyes following which a familiar object is placed in one hand. The object cannot be recognized as the same object when transferred to the other hand. Similar separation of hemispheric function can also be demonstrated in split-

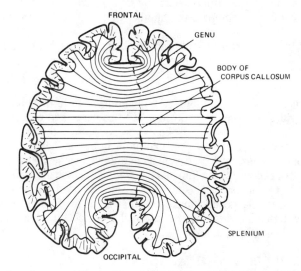

FIGURE 123. Plan view of corpus callosum. (Correlate with Figures 121, 122, and 128.)

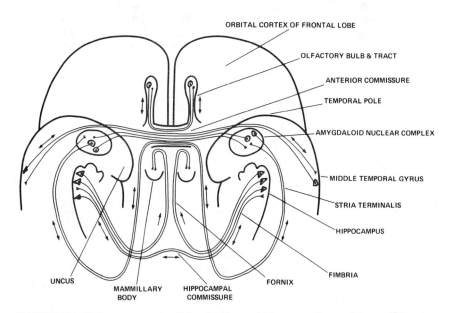

FIGURE 124. Major components of the anterior and hippocampal commissures. (Compare Figure 80.)

brain patients in the visual sphere, by taking care that the eyes do not move: the subject cannot compare the number of fingers displayed in right and left visual fields.

With intact corpus callosum, such interhemispheric correlations occur very quickly. Even here, it is possible to demonstrate a short delay between hemispheric responses, presumably due to the time required for learned information to traverse the corpus callosum.

Interestingly, split-brain individuals have little difficulty with ordinary life activities. Moving objects from hand to hand, and especially moving the eyes about so that both hemispheres receive similar though not simultaneous inputs, seems to remove the potential problem of hemispheric competition.

Under controlled experimental conditions, it appears that each hemisphere represents or mediates a completely individual personality. Each of us appears to possess two identical personalities inside the head. They are identical as a result of identical genetic make-up and identical life-long experiences, constantly correlated and mutually reinforced to perfect consonance by interactions via the corpus callosum.

CEREBRAL DOMINANCE

Nevertheless, differences exist between the functions of the two hemispheres. Left cortical lesions, particularly parietal, often cause aphasic speech difficulties. Right-sided lesions do not. This is usually correlated with right-handedness. Statistically, the left hemisphere mediates speech in all right-handed persons and about two-thirds of left-handed persons, a total of about 95 percent of persons tested.

Even before split-brain studies, observations of clinical lesions indicated differences in hemispheric functions. The left hemisphere is language-dominant, performing in symbolic spheres such as talking, reading, writing, calculations, and understanding speech, while the right hemisphere may be concerned with geometrical, geographic, structural imagery. For instance, a person with a right parietal lesion may have difficulty figuring out how to put his shirt on: which is the right sleeve? which is the top?

Clinically, lesions in the parietal or parieto-temporo-occipital cortex, particularly left-sided, often produce various types of agnosia (Greek = not know).

Dominance of the left hemisphere in speech-related symbolic functions seems to result from a combination of factors:

1. Genetic The infolded cortex of Wernicke's sensory speech area at the parietal end of the lateral fissure is broader on the left than right side in most people.

2. Cultural In most cultures, strong social pressures demand use of the right hand. The positive connotation of the word dexterous is a case in point.

3. Accidental A child with a broken arm during the speech-formative years, may change handedness, and possibly brain-sidedness.

Information in the previous paragraphs must not be applied uncritically to a child with reading or other difficulties. The child's behavior depends basically on nervous function. However, individual variability, experiences, and illnesses require a thorough understanding of more than neurological status in evaluating such children.

TABLE 15. Some specific types of agnosia

Aphasia	Inability to speak due to cortical lesion, with little or no loss of intellect.
Nominal aphasia	Inability to speak the names of objects.
Semantic aphasia	Inability to use words in proper context.
Expressive (motor) aphasia	Aphasia specifically due to lesion in Broca's area; inability to use the vocal apparatus for speech, but without paralysis or ataxia.
Receptive (sensory) aphasia	Wernicke's aphasia, speech is fluent, but often without meaning; lesion in parietal cortex.
Jargon aphasia	Aphasic replacement of normal speech by meaningless jargon. Likely to be a manifestation of receptive aphasia.
Auditory agnosia	Inability to understand or recognize spoken words.
Visual agnosia	Inability to recognize objects visually.
Astereognosis	Inability to recognize objects by feel.
Atopognosia	Inability to locate parts of the body, e.g., location of a point touched, without sensory deficit.
Right-left disorientation	Inability to distinguish right from left.
Finger agnosia	Inability to identify specific fingers
Anosognosia	Unawareness of illness; usually associated with loss of awareness of a hemiplegic limb or limbs.
Alexia	Inability to read.
Agraphia	Inability to write.
Acalculia	Inability to perform arithmetic.
Amusia	Inability to recognize or perform music.
Apraxia	Inability to perform complex movements.

CLINICAL EXAMPLE 41

A retired elevator operator, age 76, was admitted to hospital because of a stroke. He was not paralyzed, and seemed alert and intelligent. His only neurological abnormality was a right Babinski sign. On mental testing, he was unable to name common objects. A pen was recognized, as he showed by gesture, but he could not name it. His speech was usually clear, but occasionally he used words that did not fit: he said 'I went roam' instead of 'I went home,' and was nonplussed and distressed when this happened. Sometimes he could correct his verbal error.

Discussion

In a person with a probable stroke (CVA), a right Babinski sign suggests a left hemisphere lesion. This guess was supported by his nominal aphasia and mild jargon aphasia. Such disabilities often follow small vascular lesions in the left parietal cortex.

THOUGHT: THE CORTICAL PROCESS OF INTELLECTION

The almost infinite connectivity of cortical neurons must mediate the subjective experiences we call thought, memory, and reasoning, and must make up the personality. How this occurs presents the major problem of functional

In contrast to phrenological dicta, it has become apparent that no single cortical region can be assigned the functions individuality and personality. Clinical effects of multitudes of cortical lesions in tens of thousand of patients, with destruction of widely varying areas, locations, and types of cortex have clearly shown that it makes no difference which cortical area loses its function, the person retains his or her individuality, though of course specific functions may be seriously disturbed.

As Lashley concluded many years ago from studies on rats, the 'general' functions of each area of cortex are similar. Neurological and anatomical substrates of this basic similarity of function -- cortical pluripotency -- remains unclear, but some tentative comments are possible.

The multiplicity of neural interconnections appears similar in most or all cortical regions. Each neuron is potentially and indirectly connected with every other. Motor and sensory cortical representations are multiple. Perhaps we can presume that the entire personality or individuality is at least doubly represented, once in the right, once in the left hemisphere.

A clinical observation   Damage to one region of cortex usually changes the personality of the patient little. As another region, and another, and another, are damaged in sequence, as by multiple small vascular lesions (CVAs), eventually personality changes are detected. Intellectual ability gradually diminishes, memory deteriorates, and motor and sensory responsiveness decreases, leading eventually to total disintegration of the personality, usually labeled clinically as multi-infarct dementia.

HOLOGRAM ANALOGY

This kind of sequential change has suggested a hologram analogy of cortical function. A hologram is a three-dimensional photograph taken with laser light. From holographic negatives a clear three-dimensional reproduction of the original object can be obtained. Use of any half of the negative also gives an image, but not so crisp; and use of smaller fractions of any portion of the negative gives reproductions progressively less clear.

A parallel between the progressive decrease in clarity of partial holographic negatives, and the sequence of personality deterioration with repeated brain lesions is obvious. The cortex does not indeed operate like a holograph except perhaps in some mathematical sense, nevertheless the analogy seems apt and suggests a useful model of important aspects of cortical function.

The holograph analogy depends on the parallel between the almost infinite number of bits of information derived from the interference patterns between light waves of the laser, and a similar almost infinite number of cortical possibilities: 10 to 15 billion neurons, hundreds of trillions of synapses, and uncountable functional combinations. Multiply this by the variant protein structures which many feel may be involved in memory, and the number of possibilities becomes even more astronomical.

CLINICAL EXAMPLE 42

Long-term memory appears to be mediated by permanent anatomical and chemical changes in neurons and synapses. Short-term or temporary memory has not been accounted for, but some suggestions exist that memory up to 10 minutes or so may be mediated by multiple synaptic linkages. Each cubic millimeter of

*cortex includes about 1,000,000,000 (one billion) synapses, so
the anatomical substrate is clearly present. Calculate the
approximate delay that might be expected if one million synapses
within a given cubic millimeter of cortex were to act sequentially.*

Discussion

*Assuming usual synaptic delays of 0.5 to 1 msec, one million
sequential synaptic delays would sum to 500,000 to 1,000,000 msec or
8 to 16 minutes. There is, of course, no direct evidence that such
a sequential process accounts for recent memory, though the concept
is seductive. The main point of this example is to emphasize
the complexity of the cortex.*

THALAMOCORTICAL RELATIONS

Billions of axons carry action potentials from cortical areas to thalamus
and from thalamus to cortex. Some of these have been mentioned in discussion
of sensory and motor relays. Other corticothalamic connections: limbic, basal
gangliar, reticular, will be discussed later.

Beside these connections, a larger number have associational functions.
For example, numerous axons feed back from cortex to thalamus to alter
thalamic input to the cortex. More complex connections exhibit inhibitory and
excitatory effects.

Two associational bundles whose functions have been partially defined
are those connecting pulvinar and parietal cortex. Sectioning the former bundle
is frontal lobotomy or leucotomy. These fibers carry impulses through which
the individual correlates events temporally or causally. After lobotomy, the
patient is likely to be uncaring or unaware of the results of his actions. Also in
this state, his schizophrenic hallucinations no longer bother him.

The bundle connecting pulvinar and parietal cortex appears involved in
gnostic functions. Lesions of the pulvinar at times result in agnosias.

THALAMOCORTICAL ELECTROPHYSIOLOGY

Electrical relations were first defined between thalamus and cortex about
40 years ago when Morison and Dempsey demonstrated that rhythmic stimulation of the midline thalamic nuclei at certain frequencies resulted in cortical
recruitment of electroencephalographic (EEG) waves at the same frequency
(Figure 125).

Recruiting responses result from repetitive stimulation of nonspecific
thalamic nuclei, i.e., thalamic nuclei without specific motor or sensory functions. Similar responses also occur with rhythmic stimulation of specific
thalamic nuclei, but have been given the name augmenting responses.

Interactions between thalamus and cortex have much to do with the form
and frequency of the spontaneous electrical activity of the cortex, the electroencephalogram (EEG). The EEG consists of the average activity of large
numbers of cortical neurons, recorded from the surface of the scalp, directly
from the cortex, or from the depths of the brain.

Alpha activity, the most widely known EEG activity, consists of trains
of sinusoidal electrical potentials at frequencies between 8 and 12 per second,
most often about 10 per second, but specific for each individual. It commonly

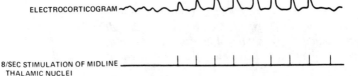

FIGURE 125. Cortical recruiting response to rhythmic stimulation of midline thalamus. The gradual increase in response amplitude is called recruitment.

appears over the parieto-occipital regions in awake relaxed adults. EEG frequencies and patterns vary over a wide range, depending on state of consciousness, age, other physiological and pathological variables, and specific individual characteristics.

Many kinds of brain pathology cause EEG abnormalities. Abnormal EEGs can provide focalizing information, or specific patterns may support specific neurological diagnoses. It is particularly useful for evaluating convulsive disorders (epilepsy), But its use extends to brain tumors, degenerative diseases, and other focal or diffuse brain pathologies.

STUDY QUESTIONS

1. Sketch a lateral view of a cerebral hemisphere, labeling major anatomical landmarks and functional areas.
2. Prepare a similar sketch of the medial view of a cerebral hemisphere.
3. What would be the clinical effect of a lesion in each of the cortical areas identified in questions 1 and 2?
4. What is meant by radial (columnar) organization of the cortex?
5. How many neurons are there in the neocortex?
6. What is meant by the point-to-point relationship between the external world and the cerebral cortex? -- Between parts of the body and the cortex? Give examples.
7. Discuss lamination of the neocortex.
8. List the possible afferent and efferent connections of cortical neurons.
9. What is the corpus callosum? What is its function?
10. What is the anterior commissure?
11. What is meant by dominant hemisphere?
12. What is agnosia? Give several examples.
13. What is meant by thalamocortical recruitment?
14. What is the EEG?
15. Describe the clinical effects of:
    a. A small lesion in area 17 on the left side.
    b. Stimulation of area 8 on the right side.
    c. Destruction of area 41 on the left side.
    d. Destruction of a large area of cortex around area 41 on the left side.
    e. Destruction of a large area of cortex around area 41 on the right side.
    f. Damage to the white matter of the frontal lobe.
    g. Cutting the corpus callosum.

13 Thalamus

Relay functions of the thalamus have been recognized for years, and have been mentioned several times in previous chapters. Lesions disturbing these parts of the thalamus cause serious neurological deficits.

Some of the other thalamic connections and functions are equally important. Particularly to be emphasized are the massive interconnections between thalamus and cortex, forming thalamocortical functional units. Two examples have been mentioned: the extensive parietal lobe connections of the pulvinar of the thalamus reflect the pulvinar's importance in speech, and probably also in certain aspects of motor function. Connections between dorsomedial nucleus of the thalamus and frontal cortex for higher intellectual functions are involved in frontal lobotomy.

GROSS APPEARANCE OF THE THALAMUS

The thalamus consists of two paired irregularly oblong collections of nuclei lying medial to the posterior limb of the internal capsule, forming most of the lateral wall of the third ventricle, part of the floor of the lateral ventricle, and overlapping the superior colliculi of the midbrain caudally (Figure 126). It can be divided grossly into three large collections of nuclei, the anterior, medial, and lateral nuclear masses, as sketched in Figures 127 and 128.

In addition, several thalamic nuclei lie within the layer of myelinated axons, the internal medullary lamina, separating medial from lateral nuclear masses. Of these intralaminar nuclei, the centrum medianum is the largest, and is anatomically useful as a landmark for the sensory relay nuclei VPL and VPM (Figures 127, 129, and 134).

Sensory relay nuclei discussed in previous chapters include:

VPL: ventral posterolateral; somatosensory via medial lemniscus from contralateral body.

VPM: ventral posteromedial; somatosensory via trigeminal lemniscus from contralateral face. VPL and VPM together are often referred to as the ventrobasal complex.

LGB: lateral geniculate body; vision via optic tract from contralateral visual field (of both eyes — review Figure 88).

MGB: medial geniculate body; hearing via inferior quadrigeminal brachium from the inferior colliculus. LGB, MGB, and pulvinar may be grouped as the posterior thalamus.

All these nuclei also lie within the lateral nuclear mass. The lateral-ventral nucleus receives inputs from the dentate nucleus of the cerebellum via the superior cerebellar peduncle (brachium conjunctivum). Anteroventral nucleus receives most of its inputs from the globus pallidus via the ansa lenticularis, as discussed in the next chapter (see Figure 129).

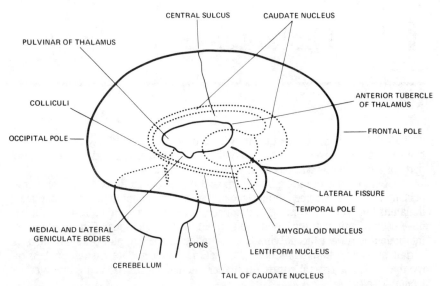

FIGURE 126. Lateral phantom sketch to show location of thalamus and other deep nuclei within the cerebral hemisphere. (Compare Figure 132 B and C.)

Afferents to lateral-ventral and anteroventral nuclei overlap to some degree. Both nuclei send their efferent axons via internal capsule to the motor cortex, areas 4 and 6, with some fibers to the somatosensory cortex.

Relays for the limbic system pass via the anterior nuclear mass, which receives inputs from the mammillary body of the hypothalamus of the same side via the mammillothalamic tract (Figures 128 and 129). Mammillary bodies in turn receive inputs from the hippocampus in the depths of the temporal lobe by way of the fornix, and from other hypothalamic and reticular neurons.

From anterior nuclei, fibers project through the anterior limb of the internal capsule to the cortex of the cingulate gyrus.

Also with major limbic connections is the dorsomedial nucleus and some of the other nuclei of the medial nuclear mass. The dorsomedial nucleus is reciprocally connected with anterior hypothalamus, with limbic system structures of the frontal and temporal lobes, and with the frontal cortex itself. These frontal connections are severed in the operation of frontal lobotomy.

Functional correlates of these connections suggest a simplified plan of the thalamic components, as sketched in Figure 130. The anterior nuclear mass and most of the medial nuclear mass are limbic structures (discussed in Chapter 17). The rostral part of the lateral nuclear mass contains neurons with motor functions. Its occipital part is mostly sensory. Pulvinar and associated nuclei seem concerned with integration for a variety of sensory and motor functions such as the gnosis mentioned in the previous chapter, and has therefore been called 'multimodal'. Finally, intralaminar nuclei and some of the nuclei of the medial nuclear mass have 'nonspecific' functions, particularly related to the brainstem reticular formation.

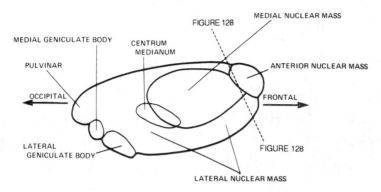

FIGURE 127. Lateral view of the thalamus. (Correlate with Figures 126 and 128.)

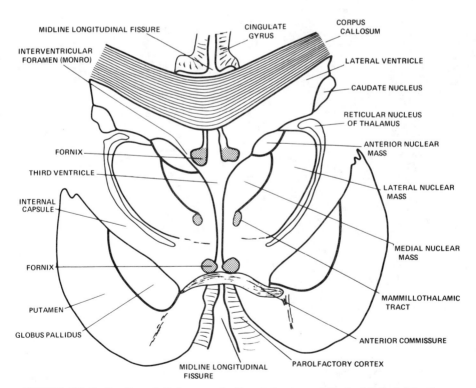

FIGURE 128. Section through thalamus and adjacent structures at the level indicated by the dashed line of Figure 127.

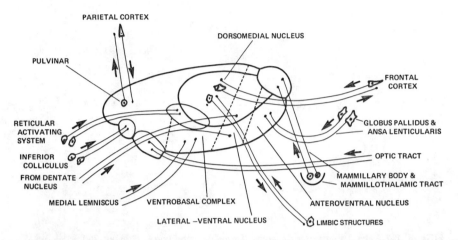

FIGURE 129. Some major connections of thalamic nuclei. The ventrobasal complex includes the ventral posterolateral and ventral posteromedial nuclei (VPL and VPM). (Correlate with Figure 127.)

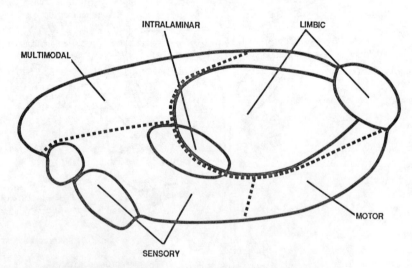

FIGURE 130. Major functional subdivisions of the human thalamus. (Correlate with Figure 129.)

NONSPECIFIC PROJECTION NUCLEI

Stimulation of the reticular activating system (RAS) of the midbrain (Figures 129 and 131) causes the EEG to lose most of its resting alpha activity, leaving low-voltage fast beta activity. Simultaneously, there is behavioral arousal; alerting if awake, awakening if asleep.

Ascending axons from the RAS enter the thalamus from below to terminate in neurons of the nonspecific projection nuclei, which include centrum medianum and other intralaminar nuclei, and some of the midline nuclei of the medial nuclear mass.

From these nonspecific projection nuclei, impulses relayed from the RAS pass further rostrally to the orbital cortex of the frontal lobe thence to the entire cortex of the same side. The RAS straddles the midline, and activates nonspecific thalamic nuclei of both sides, each of which in turn activates the ipsilateral cerebral cortex.

As discussed earlier in the chapter on sensory mechanisms, a relay from midline nuclei to orbital cortex is believed to mediate the primitive unlocalized type of pain. Section of these fibers by an inferior frontal lobotomy may be helpful to patients with intractable pain. Such patients report that the pain, previously unendurable, is still present but not bothersome.

Draped like a blanket between lateral nuclear mass and internal capsule, the reticular nucleus (Figures 128 and 134) was originally believed to be a relay nucleus, as it relates point-to-point with ipsilateral cortex. The reticular nucleus of the thalamus (*note* to be clearly distinguished from the reticular formation of the midbrain) appear to be an intermediary between cortex and thalamus, relaying inputs from the cortex on to thalamic nuclei in a point-to-point fashion. These relays seem to mediate cortical inhibition of some aspects of thalamic function.

In addition to their specific functions, most thalamic nuclei perform in thalamo-cortical integrative circuits. They project axons to the cortex (ending in layer IV) and receive axons from layer VI of the same cortical areas. Intrathalamic circuits are also complex, some concerned with sharpening incoming sensory impulses by lateral inhibition, others in organizing motor relays, others in controlling the EEG, and many with functions not yet defined.

CLINICAL EXAMPLE 43

An elderly gentleman was brought to the hospital in coma, after what his family described as a stroke. He responded only slightly and nonspecifically when stimulated on any of his four extremities, body, or face. He was able to move all four extremities and his face. The only other abnormality was an enlarged right pupil which did not react to light. Where was the lesion?

Discussion

The cerebral cortex is the organ of consciousness, whence coma implies either a diffuse cortical lesion or a lesion of the reticular activating system. Absence of paralysis (he could move all extremities) suggests that cortical functions were intact, as does his response to sensory stimulation.

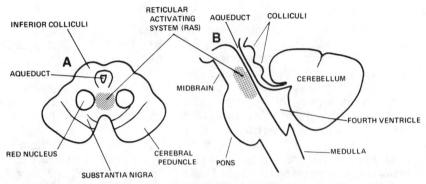

FIGURE 131. Location of the reticular activating system (RAS) within midbrain and upper pontine tegmentum in transverse (A) and midsagittal (B) sections through the region.

Unresponsiveness and mydriasis of the right pupil indicates a lesion of the right III nerve. Inasmuch as oculomotor nerve fibers exit ventrally through the RAS of the midbrain, this combination of findings can best be accounted for by a lesion, probably vascular, in the RAS of the right midbrain tegmentum. (See Figures 78, 79, and 131).

CLINICAL EXAMPLE 44

Over two months, a 45-year-old man developed loss of sensation of his entire right side. This was followed by gradually developing ataxia of the right arm, then progressively decreasing level of consciousness, culminating in coma. A radioactive brain scan showed a hot spot in the left thalamic region, strongly suggesting a brain tumor. How might such a lesion account for the findings?

Discussion

Gradual loss of right-sided sensation suggests progressive destruction of the sensory relay systems of the left thalamus. The ataxia may be the result of invasion of cerebellar relays from dentate nucleus to lateral-ventral and anteroventral nuclei. Obtundation progressing to coma suggests that the tumor grew into and destroyed the projection pathways from the RAS, or perhaps it grew into the RAS itself.

STUDY QUESTIONS

1. Name the sensory relay nuclei of the thalamus and the sensory modalities they relay.
2. Name the motor relay nuclei of the thalamus and their major afferent and efferent connections.
3. What is the thalamic syndrome? (Clinical Example 17).
4. Describe the process of lateral inhibition as it occurs in the thalamus.
5. Where is the seat of consciousness?
6. What is the internal capsule?
7. What are the intralaminar nuclei of the thalamus?

14 Basal Ganglia

In the depths of the cerebral hemispheres are several large collections of neurons, the basal ganglia, derived embryologically from the lower lip of the telencephalic vesicle. Phylogenetically, they count among the oldest of the forebrain nuclei. In some species, they constitute the highest motor control centers. In humans they also have motor functions, though additional functions have been suggested for the more recent evolutionary acquisitions.

The major nuclei of the basal ganglia are the relatively old globus pallidus (paleostriatum) and the newer caudate nucleus and putamen (neostriatum).

Often included with the basal ganglia, several nontelencephalic nuclei concerned with motor functions include the subthalamic nucleus and zona incerta in the subthalamic region (diencephalon), and the substantia nigra in the midbrain (mesencephalon).

Because all these nuclei lie outside the pyramidal tract, and subsume motor functions, their clinical malfunctions are commonly labeled extrapyramidal diseases.

GROSS APPEARANCE OF THE BASAL GANGLIA

Figures 132 and 134 show the location of the lentiform nucleus (globus pallidus plus putamen) lateral to the internal capsule, and deep to the insula in the depths of the lateral fissure. In Figures 50B and 62B, horizontal sections through the cerebrum show the relations between lentiform nucleus, caudate nucleus, thalamus, and internal capsule. In Figures 50C, 62C, and 79, midbrain cross-sections indicate locations of red nucleus and substantia nigra. Figures 128, 132, and 134 are standard sections through the cerebrum to show these relationships in somewhat more detail.

MAJOR CONNECTIONS OF THE BASAL GANGLIA

Caudate nucleus and putamen derive from a single primordium, the striatum (also called neostriatum). They receive topographically organized inputs from wide areas of cortex, including motor and association cortex, and project principally to globus pallidus which is the main outflow nucleus of the basal ganglia. The caudate nucleus has important inputs from prefrontal cortex, and from the substantia nigra of the midbrain. This latter connection is a large dopamine-carrying bundle involved in the pathology of Parkinson's disease.

Most efferents from the globus pallidus form the ansa lenticularis (Figures 132C and 133). The ansa consists of axons which exit the pallidum and loop medially around the ventral face of the internal capsule, then tend caudally between the zona incerta dorsally and the subthalamic nucleus ventrally. Some of the fibers end in these nuclei. Others continue caudally to the

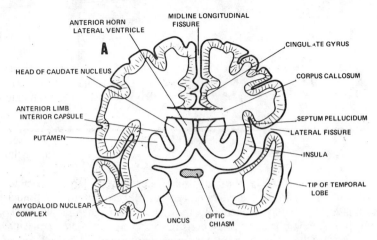

A

MIDLINE LONGITUDINAL FISSURE

ANTERIOR HORN LATERAL VENTRICLE

CINGULATE GYRUS

HEAD OF CAUDATE NUCLEUS

CORPUS CALLOSUM

ANTERIOR LIMB INTERIOR CAPSULE

SEPTUM PELLUCIDUM

PUTAMEN

LATERAL FISSURE

INSULA

TIP OF TEMPORAL LOBE

AMYGDALOID NUCLEAR COMPLEX

UNCUS

OPTIC CHIASM

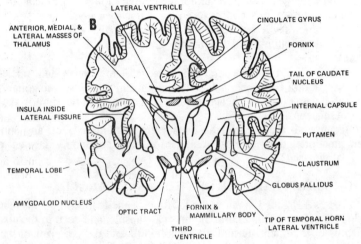

B

LATERAL VENTRICLE

ANTERIOR, MEDIAL, & LATERAL MASSES OF THALAMUS

CINGULATE GYRUS

FORNIX

TAIL OF CAUDATE NUCLEUS

INSULA INSIDE LATERAL FISSURE

INTERNAL CAPSULE

PUTAMEN

CLAUSTRUM

TEMPORAL LOBE

GLOBUS PALLIDUS

AMYGDALOID NUCLEUS

OPTIC TRACT

FORNIX & MAMMILLARY BODY

THIRD VENTRICLE

TIP OF TEMPORAL HORN LATERAL VENTRICLE

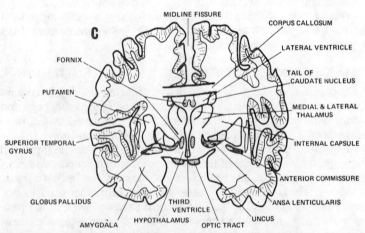

C

MIDLINE FISSURE

CORPUS CALLOSUM

LATERAL VENTRICLE

FORNIX

TAIL OF CAUDATE NUCLEUS

PUTAMEN

MEDIAL & LATERAL THALAMUS

SUPERIOR TEMPORAL GYRUS

INTERNAL CAPSULE

ANTERIOR COMMISSURE

GLOBUS PALLIDUS

ANSA LENTICULARIS

THIRD VENTRICLE

AMYGDALA

HYPOTHALAMUS

OPTIC TRACT

UNCUS

FIGURE 132. Coronal sections through basal ganglia. The sections are from different brains, therefore not completely comparable. They are asymmetrical because of imperfectly transverse cuts. In (C) the ansa lenticularis can be seen leaving the globus pallidus and looping ventrally around the internal capsule on its way to the AV thalamus.

red nucleus, the substantia nigra, or further, as the central tegmental tract to brain stem reticular formation and inferior olivary nucleus (Figures 75-77).

Many of the fibers loop backward, then rostrally between the zona incerta and the under surface of the thalamus to terminate in the anteroventral (AV) nucleus of the thalamus. A few fibers go to the lateral-ventral (LV) nucleus. Both AV and LV relay to motor cortex areas 4 and 6. Some of these fibers go to the centrum medianum of the thalamus (one of the intralaminar nuclei — see Figures 127 and 134), whence they relay back to the striatum.

As they loop around the zona incerta, these fibers are called fields of Forel. Field H2 are the fibers between zona incerta and subthalamic nucleus. Field H refers to fibers between zona incerta and red nucleus. Field H1 lies between zona incerta and thalamus. Three other synonyms are occasionally seen:

> Field H1: Fasciculus thalamicus
> Field H: Prerubral field
> Field H2: Fasciculus lenticularis.

BASAL GANGLIAR FEEDBACK LOOPS

As in many neural situations, feedback loops are important in the organization and function of the basal ganglia. The most important loop arises from many cortical areas, feeding excitation into caudate nucleus and putamen (neostriatum). Within the neostriatum, acetylcholinergic neurons excited by the cortical input in turn excite a GABA inhibitory outflow to the globus pallidus. From the globus pallidus, the ansa lenticularis transmits excitation to anteroventral and lateral-ventral thalamus, which relay excitation to cells of origin of the pyramidal tract in motor cortex areas 4 and 6 (see Figure 135).

Subsidiary to this major cortex-to-cortex loop are two others. The best known sends excitatory and inhibitory impulses from neostriatum to substantia nigra. From the substantia nigra dopamine-carrying axons return to the neostriatum, where each axon terminates in inhibitory synapses on about 500,000 neurons. This is the loop which is disrupted in Parkinson's disease.

The second loop goes from globus pallidus to form excitatory terminals in the subthalamic nucleus, followed by an inhibitory feedback from the subthalamic nucleus. Lesions here cause ballism (Figure 135).

FUNCTIONS OF BASAL GANGLIA: EFFECTS OF LESIONS

Detailed and specific functions of individual basal ganglia have not yet been defined. They operate principally in the motor sphere, through connections just discussed. However, most current knowledge of function comes from analysis of numerous clinical lesions of the structures.

Lesions in the substantia nigra with secondary changes in globus pallidus commonly occur in patients with paralysis agitans (Parkinson's disease). This clinicopathologic correlation has been shown in recent years to relate to the nigrostriatal dopaminergic system, mentioned earlier. Substantia nigra (Latin = black substance) is so named after the numerous melanin-containing neurons in the nucleus. These neurons elaborate dopamine which their axons transfer to the caudate nucleus and putamen. In Parkinson's disease, the pigment-containing neurons degenerate, the substantia nigra loses its black color, and the caudate and putamen lose their dopamine input.

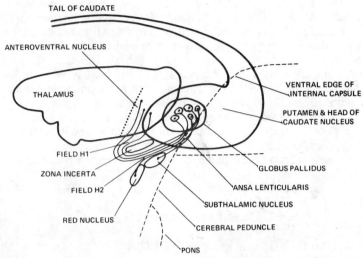

FIGURE 133. Lateral phantom sketch to show the circuitous pathway of the ansa lenticularis from the globus pallidus to the anteroventral thalamus.

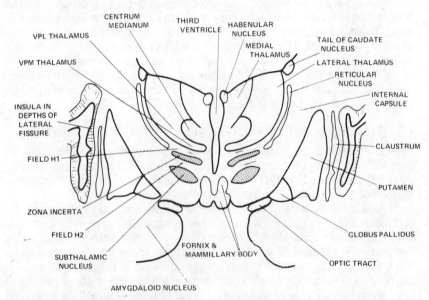

FIGURE 134. Coronal section through basal ganglia at the level of subthalamic nucleus. (Compare Figures 132 and 133.)

Treatment of Parkinsonian patients with L-dopa (L-dihydroxyphenylala-nine), the immediate precursor of dopamine, may greatly improve their motor defects, presumably by supplying the neurotransmitter to caudate and putamen.

Lesions of the lentiform nucleus commonly give rise to contralateral dyskinesia (abnormal involuntary movement) of three overlapping types:

1. **Chorea:** sudden, twitching, involuntary movements.

2. **Athetosis:** slower, writhing or worm-like involuntary movements.

3. **Dystonia:** sustained postural contractions of limb, neck, or facial muscles.

These three types of dyskinesia differ clinically only in their rapidity. A slow-motion picture of a choreatic patient looks athetotic, and vice-versa. The exact differences between various lesions to induce these different dyskinesias are unknown.

Lesions in the subthalamic nucleus cause another type of dyskinesia called ballism, or hemiballism if present only on one side. These are violent, throwing (Greek, ballein = throw) movements of an entire arm or leg.

Parkinson's disease, whose primary lesion is in the substantia nigra, includes dyskinetic muscle contractions of two types: pill-rolling tremor and rigidity. The tremor is named after the finger movement formerly used by pharmacists to prepare pills by hand. Rigidity means constant contraction of muscles. Because of the constant contraction, the patient's movement slows or may become impossible. Gait stiffens; the patient has difficulty keeping up with his center of gravity. The patient walks in small steps because of his rigidity, but has to walk faster to prevent falling. This is the festinating gait (Latin = hurry). These patients also have a mask-like face, partially because of rigidity of facial muscles. Akinesia or difficulty initiating movement is also commonly part of the syndrome.

Liver disease often causes brain damage, more commonly to basal ganglia than elsewhere. Wilson's disease (hepatolenticular degeneration) is the classical type; it results from faulty copper metabolism. Patients with liver disease often demonstrate a distinctive postural dyskinesia called asterixis or liver flap. With arm extended, the patient's wrist extensors involuntarily relax, causing a hand movement like 'waving goodbye.'

Blood incompatibilities, such as Rh type, between mother and fetus may cause erythroblastosis fetalis with blood cell destruction, liver damage, and damage to the basal ganglia, which become discolored by the blood pigments. This condition may be called by its German name, kernicterus.

CLINICAL EXAMPLE 45

A gentleman, 57 years old, developed a right-sided pill-rolling tremor,
a mild festinating gait, some rigidity of the right arm and leg, and
did not swing his right arm when walking. A lesion was produced
by stereotaxic surgery in the left LV thalamus, following which
his rigidity improved, and the tremor decreased somewhat.

Discussion

The findings listed are characteristic of right-sided Parkinson's
disease (paralysis agitans). LV thalamus relays basal ganglia outflow

TABLE 16. Signs of various lesions of human motor systems

Location of lesion	Voluntary strength	Atrophy	Muscle stretch reflexes	Tone	Abnormal movements	Electrical findings
Muscle (1) (myopathy)	Weak (2) (paretic)	Present	Hypoactive	Hypotonic	None	Small MUAP (9)
Motor endplate (MEP), (myasthenia)	Paretic	None	Hypoactive	Hypotonic	None	Fatigable
LMN (including peripheral nerve: neuropathy	Paretic	Severe	Hypoactive	Hypotonic	Fasciculations (5)	Fibrillations (10) small or large MUAP
UMN	Paretic or or plegic (2)	Mild (disuse)	Hyperactive (spastic) (3) (11)	Hypertonic 'clasp knife'	Withdrawal spasms (Babinski) (6)	Normal MUAP
Cerebellar systems	Normal	None	Normal	Hypotonic (4) (pendulous)	Ataxia dysmetria	Normal MUAP
Basal ganglia	Normal	None	Normal	Rigid: 'lead pipe'	Dyskinesia (7)	Normal MUAP, spontaneous contractions
Cortical association areas	Usually normal	Usually none	Normal or spastic	Usually normal	Apraxia (8)	Normal MUAP

(1) Myopathies are degenerative processes involving muscle fibers directly.

(2) Weak = paretic; paralyzed = plegic.

(3) Hyperactive reflexes = hyperreflexia = spasticity.

(4) Hypotonic because of decreased activation of gamma efferent system.

(5) Fasciculations are spontaneous contractions of entire motor units. They cause grossly visible twitches. Contrast with (10).

(6) Babinski reflex = extensor plantar response is a partial withdrawal reflex, a spinal phenomenon released from suprasegmental control.

(7) Such as chorea, athetosis, dystonia, rest tremors, ballism, asterixis.

(8) Apraxia = motor agnosia. Cortical integrative or organizing mechanisms for normal movements are defective.

(9) MUAP = motor unit action potential.

(10) Fibrillations = contractions of single muscle fibers, usually the result of denervation. Not visible grossly; detectable only with electrical (electromyogram = EMG) recording.

(11) Following an acute UMN lesion, reflexes are often absent (hypoactive) for a period of days or weeks. This condition is called 'spinal or cerebral shock.'

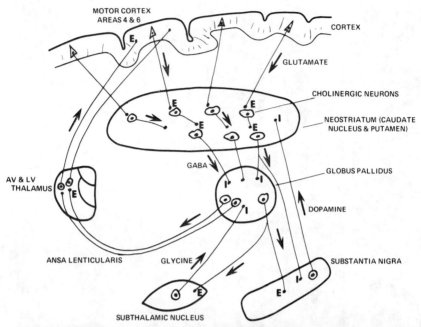

FIGURE 135. Diagram showing some basal gangliar connections. In particular note the three major feedback loops described in the text. (I) and (E) indicate inhibitory and excitatory synapses, respectively.

to the motor cortex. No adequate explanation has yet been supplied for the improvement which may follow destructive lesions here, globus pallidus, or in the ansa lenticularis. Evidently, the damaged basal ganglia produce abnormal patterns of motor control. Their removal by lesioning cannot return the patient to normal, but at least decreases the abnormal input into the motor cortex.

CLINICAL EXAMPLE 46

A boy of 10 years had had a flu-like illness the month before, and was brought in because he was twitchy and nervous, seeming unable to sit still. On examination, his face and both arms twitched irregularly and without voluntary control. A diagnosis of Sydenham's infectious chorea was made, the flu apparently having been the causative illness. Where was the lesion?

Discussion

The lesion was within the basal ganglia, probably the result of rheumatic (i.e., atopic) disease associated with the flu. The chorea is usually temporary, and immediate prognosis is exellent. Unfortunately, permanent basal gangliar damage may occur, leaving long-term effects. Also, the possibility must be kept in mind that the heart or other organs may have been damaged.

CLINICAL EXAMPLE 47

A man with Parkinson's disease reported that at times he would burst into tears or laughter without any reason. This was exceedingly embarrassing. The episodes occurred less often under L-dopa treatment. Discuss.

Discussion

Spontaneous laughter or crying occur in certain patients with Parkinson's disease. These are dissociated motor manifestations of emotion — emotional motor activity without emotional feeling. The phenomenon may be related to the mask-like face of these patients. Probably this kind of spontaneous content-free pseudo-emotional reaction results from damage to the ventral tegmental nucleus, a dopaminergic limbic system nucleus which lies adjacent to the substantia nigra and projects to rostral limbic system structures and cortex. Disturbances of the function of limbic system components probably accounted for the patient's pathological pseudo-emotional manifestations.

CLINICAL EXAMPLE 48

An elderly gentleman with known hypertension suffered a stroke following which his right arm would, at regular intervals, fling wildly to the side. These movements were involuntary, and not under conscious control. In desperation, the patient constantly maintained a firm grip on his right arm with his left hand to avoid hurting himself as his arm flailed about. Where was the lesion?

Discussion

Wild, 'throwing' involuntary movements of this nature are called ballism — or more accurately, since only one side was involved, hemiballism. This gentleman's right-sided hemiballism resulted from a vascular lesion of the left subthalamic nucleus.

STUDY QUESTIONS

1. Name the basal ganglia and give their locations.
2. Name the principal inputs and outputs of the basal ganglia.
3. What is meant by dyskinesia?
4. Define: Chorea; Athetosis; Dystonia; Pill-rolling tremor; Rigidity; Mask-like face; Festinating gait; Ballism; Asterixis.
5. What would you expect to be the result of cutting the pyramidal tract on the motor manifestations of Parkinson's disease? (For a time this was tried therapeutically.)

15 Autonomic Nervous System

Those portions of the central and peripheral nervous systems which control involuntary body functions make up the autonomic nervous system (ANS). Such functions are usually labeled visceral, meaning the control of smooth muscle in thoracic and abdominal viscera, in the eye, in blood vessels, and in the skin, as well as control of exocrine (but not endocrine) glands, and control of the heart rate. Visceral efferent or visceromotor are terms commonly used to refer to these systems. Although the heart consists of striated muscle, it is not under direct voluntary control as are other striated muscles.

All of these functions serve to maintain the body's physicochemical equilibrium, a general concept called homeostasis. Implied are constant temperature, constant electrolyte concentrations, maintenance of nutrients in the blood, and maintenance of blood flow, with variations as demanded by momentary needs of organs. Included also are the processes of assimilation and elimination, and the preservation of the individual and the species.

The two major divisions of the ANS, as charted in Table 17, can be functionally related to their effects on homeostasis.

SYMPATHETIC NERVOUS SYSTEM (SNS)

Sympathetic neurons in the CNS lie in the lateral horn of the spinal cord, mostly in the thoracic and upper lumbar segments. Their white myelinated ventral root fibers leave the spinal nerve just outside the intervertebral foramen (Figure 136) as the white ramus, going to the sympathetic chain of ganglia, the paravertebral ganglia. These fibers are designated preganglionic, because their first synapse outside the CNS occurs in the sympathetic ganglia.

The sympathetic chain consists of a paired linear series of 22 or 23 ganglia with longitudinal interconnecting fibers, one chain lying on either side of the vertebral bodies from midcervical region to the coccyx. Three cervical

TABLE 17. Major subdivisions of the autonomic nervous system

Division of ANS	Locations	General functions	Neurotransmitter
Sympathetic nervous system (SNS)	Thoracolumbar T1 to L2 (lateral horn)	Fight, fright, or flight	Norepinephrine. (Adrenalin from adrenal gland; acetylcholine to sweat glands)
Parasympathetic nervous system (PSNS)	Craniosacral: cranial nerves III, VII, IX, X: sacral 2-4	Rest, recuperation, and reproduction	Acetylcholine

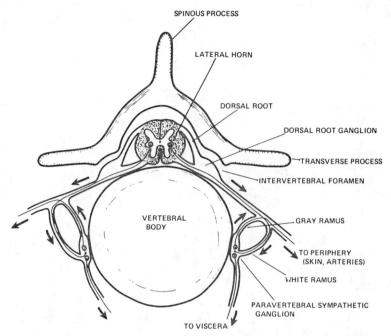

SPINOUS PROCESS

LATERAL HORN

DORSAL ROOT

DORSAL ROOT GANGLION

TRANSVERSE PROCESS

INTERVERTEBRAL FORAMEN

VERTEBRAL BODY

GRAY RAMUS

TO PERIPHERY (SKIN, ARTERIES)

WHITE RAMUS

PARAVERTEBRAL SYMPATHETIC GANGLION

TO VISCERA

FIGURE 136. Major sympathetic connections from the lateral horn of the spinal cord. Peripheral fibers supply sweat glands, arrectors of hair, and arteries of skin and muscle. (Compare Figures 6, 7, 8, and 137.)

ganglia, 10 or 11 thoracic ganglia, four lumbar ganglia, four sacral ganglia, and one coccygeal ganglion make up each chain. The inferior cervical ganglion often fuses with the T1 ganglion to form the large stellate ganglion (Figure 137).

White rami connect the sympathetic chain with spinal nerves at each thoracic level and the upper two lumbar levels, gray rami at all levels. Cervical sympathetic ganglia receive inputs via fibers ascending the chain from upper thoracic levels. Lower lumbar and sacral ganglia receive fibers descending the chain from lower thoracic or upper lumbar levels.

Within the chain of ganglia, preganglionic fibers synapse with SNS neurons in ganglia at the same, higher, or lower levels. After integrative processes involving dopaminergic interneurons, they send postganglionic axons either back to the spinal nerves as gray rami (gray because unmyelinated), or to prevertebral plexuses or ganglia in the abdominal cavity. Some preganglionic fibers traverse the chain without synapsing, continuing to the prevertebral ganglia where they synapse, and postganglionic fibers supply abdominal viscera.

Postganglionic fibers affect the viscera in various ways. They speed the heart rate, dilate the bronchioles of the lungs, slow down or stop peristalsis of stomach and intestines, and constrict pyloric, iloececal and rectal sphincters. All these events ready the body as a whole for emergency activity (see 'fight, fright, and flight' in Table 17).

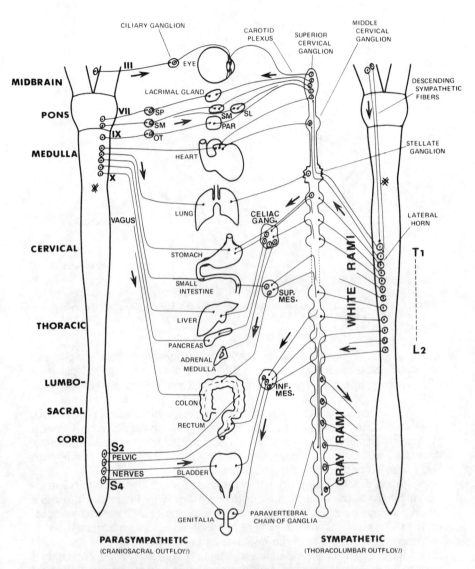

FIGURE 137. Pattern of autonomic innervation; sympathetic summarized to right, parasympathetic to left. III, VII, and X refer to cranial nerves.

SP = Sphenopalatine ganglion	SM = Submaxillary ganglion and gland
SL = Sublingual gland	PAR = Parotid gland
OT = Otic ganglion	SUP.MES = Superior mesenteric ganglion
INF.MES = Inferior mesenteric ganglion (prevertebral)	

White rami occur segmentally from T1 to L2; gray rami occur at all levels, but are sketched here only at lumbosacral levels for simplification.

Glandular effects are similar. Digestive glands generally are turned off, and the adrenal medulla secretes epinephrine (adrenalin) and some norepinephrine into the blood stream. Peripherally, the SNS causes dilation of blood vessels to somatic muscle, increasing the muscle's source of energy, but constriction of dermal blood vessels, resulting in blanching of the skin and also shunting more blood to the muscles.

Structures of the head receive their sympathetic input from the superior cervical ganglion. These impulses cause mydriasis of the pupil, secretion of viscous mucous saliva (as in the dry mouth of nervousness or fright), constriction of small arteries of the face to cause blanching, and pilo-erection (hair standing on end). Postganglionic fibers from the superior cervical ganglion travel with the carotid artery as the carotid plexus, following arterial branches and other nerves to the structures supplied. As mentioned in the discussion of Horner's syndrome (page 106) central SNS fibers descend the ipsilateral brain stem from hypothalamus to T1 for the control of pupillary dilation.

Sympathetic supply to the heart and lungs arises from the upper five thoracic segments, preganglionic fibers pass rostrally in the chain to the middle or inferior cervical ganglia, then postganglionic fibers descend into the thorax as cardiac nerves to supply heart and lungs.

In many instances, SNS activity effects a 'mass discharge,' i.e., changes in blood vessels of skin and muscles, activation of sweat glands, tachycardia, dilation of bronchioles, slowing of peristalsis, and other effects all occur simultaneously.

PARASYMPATHETIC NERVOUS SYSTEM (PSNS)

Parasympathetic preganglionic fibers are generally much longer and postganglionic fibers much shorter than the sympathetic. PSNS preganglionic fibers travel to their first synapse in ganglia which lie close to or inside the innervated organ.

For example, the PSNS fibers from oculomotor nucleus mediating pupilloconstriction synapse first in the ciliary ganglion just behind the eyeball. Some go further to episcleral ganglia in the wall of the eyeball itself (Figures 92 and 137). From these parasympathetic ganglia, postganglionic fibers are very short, in contrast with the long, sympathetic postganglionic fibers from the superior cervical ganglion.

PSNS fibers of the VII facial nerve originate from the small superior salivatory nucleus in the medulla (Figure 73). They leave the main facial nerve within the petrous bone as the chorda tympani and the greater superficial petrosal nerve. The former, which also bears taste fibers, has its first synapse in the submaxillary ganglion under the floor of the mouth. Postganglionic fibers then innervate the sublingual and submaxillary salivary glands. In contrast to the sparse mucous secretion induced by SNS stimulation, the PSNS evokes a profuse watery, serous secretion, for effective moistening of food being chewed.

Fibers of the greater superficial petrosal nerve go to the sphenopalatine ganglion. Postganglionic fibers accompany branches of the trigeminal (V) cranial nerve to the lacrimal gland in the lateral orbit, where they cause secretion of tears.

PSNS fibers in the glossopharyngeal (IX) nerve arise from the inferior salivatory nucleus in the medulla. They synapse in the otic ganglion just medial to the ear on the base of the skull, and short postganglionic fibers innervate the large parotid gland at the angle of the jaw. This gland becomes swollen and painful in mumps.

In the caudal floor of the fourth ventricle, the dorsal motor nucleus of the vagus is the most prominent PSNS nucleus. It lies just caudal to the salivatory nuclei. PSNS fibers of the vagus (Latin = wandering) follow a long course down the neck into thoracic cavity to heart and lungs, then into the abdominal cavity to innervate smooth muscles and glands in stomach, intestines, and other viscera.

These nerves generally oppose actions of the SNS. They activate peristalsis and the secretion of digestive enzymes. They act to support digestion of food, and the building-up of body energy stores.

Scattered neurons in the central portion of the gray matter of sacral 2-3-4 make up the sacral PSNS. Their axons exit via ventral roots, and form a plexus in the pelvis from which pelvic nerves extend distally to innervate the urinary bladder and genitalia (Figure 137).

This combination of effects justifies the phrase 'rest, recuperation, and reproduction' of Table 17. In additional contrast to the mass effect common with SNS activation, the PSNS most often results in effects which tend to be isolated to one organ or system.

MICTURITION, SEXUAL FUNCTION, AND PERISTALSIS

Sacral PSNS fibers, together with SNS fibers from lower thoracic and upper lumbar levels via splanchnic nerve and the hypogastric presacral plexus, control the act of micturition (urination) and the complex events which make up sexual arousal and ejaculation. The SNS appears to inhibit bladder contraction and constrict the external sphincter, preventing urination.

In contrast, the PSNS relaxes the external sphincter and induces contraction of the detrusor muscle of the bladder to force urine out of the bladder, with added pressure from voluntary straining of abdominal muscles.

Sexual reflex afferents originate from glans and adjacent skin and mucous membranes. The fibers enter the cord at S2-3-4, then after synaptic interaction, impulses return via the pelvic nerves to the genitalia to cause erection and secretion from accessory glands. This appears mainly a PSNS function, but some feel that the SNS plays important roles. Higher centers are also important, influencing the events via impulses descending the length of the spinal cord.

In the walls of the hollow viscera (esophagus, stomach, intestines, urinary bladder, gall bladder), intrinsic nervous plexuses, called Auerbach's and Meissner's in the gut, receive and respond to ANS inputs. These plexuses consist of ganglion cells and diffuse networks of unmyelinated nerve fibers which give the gastrointestinal tube a degree of autonomy, with relatively normal function even when all external neural inputs have been removed. Once started by the voluntary act of swallowing, peristalsis may continue as the intrinsic nerve networks transmit nerve impulses inducing contractions from one segment of gut to the next, forcing the bolus of food along.

PSNS inputs increase the rate and force of peristaltic movements, SNS inputs inhibit them.

NEUROTRANSMITTERS

Acetylcholine (ACh) is the neurotransmitter at preganglionic synapses, both PSNS and SNS. Most postganglionic PSNS synapses secrete ACh. Most postganglionic SNS synapses use norepinephrine, but SNS effectors that induce sweating and vasodilation in somatic muscle use ACh.

Somatic muscle motor endplates also utilize ACh. It has different effects in these three situations, however, because of differences in the postsynaptic receptor molecules. These differences become important in pharmacology, where the effects of drugs in many instances depend on their actions on ACh receptors. In fact, the dichotomy of ACh synapses into two general types is derived from their reactions to the drugs nicotine and muscarine. Nicotinic endings include preganglionic ACh synapses and somatic motor endplates. These in turn can be distinguished by the observation that hexamethonium paralyzes the former and curare the latter. Muscarinic ACh synapses include those controlling smooth muscle and glands, and they are paralyzed by atropine. Norepinephrine synapses also have two types of postsynaptic receptor molecules, alpha or beta. Alpha-adrenergic endings (responding to norepinephrine or epinephrine) include those involved in vasoconstriction, pupillodilation, and gastrointestinal sphincter constriction. Beta-adrenergic endings cause vasodilation, bronchodilation, decreased intestinal motility, and increased heart rate.

Adrenalin (epinephrine) and about one-fourth as much norepinephrine are secreted by the adrenal medulla in response to SNS stimulation (Figure 137). This effect on the adrenal and its exciting effect on the body was known long before the discovery of norepinephrine; even before the mechanisms of chemical synaptic function were understood. The adrenal medulla can be thought of as a giant synapse, with epinephrine as its neurotransmitter, and with the entire body in the postsynaptic locus through the intermediary of the blood. Adrenal gland activity is a major mediator of the SNS mass effect mentioned earlier.

CENTRAL AUTONOMIC REFLEXES

Several central autonomic reflexes are important in clinical diagnosis or treatment, and in the maintenance of homeostasis.

VOMITING REFLEX

Impulses arise from the vomiting center in the reticular formation of the floor of the fourth ventricle to cause vomiting. These impulses pass into the nearby parasympathetic dorsal motor nucleus of the vagus, and via reticulospinal tracts, to the sympathetic lateral horns of thoracic spinal cord, to stop peristalsis and relax the cardiac (upper) sphincter of the stomach. At the same time descending influences stimulate anterior horn motoneurons at thoracic and lumbar levels to initiate strong reflex contraction of intercostal and abdominal muscles, expelling stomach contents.

Stimulation of the vomiting center may be direct, as with certain drugs such as apomorphine. It may also be initiated via vestibular inputs as in motion sickness.

Nauseating smells also may induce vomiting, probably by direct connections from brain stem olfactory centers. Even cortical inputs can cause vomiting. Vomiting is most important, however, in the removal of irritant materials from the stomach, the afferent limb or the reflex traveling directly to the medulla up the vagus nerve or via visceral afferent inputs to the spinal cord.

CAROTID SINUS

Blood pressure stimulates the carotid sinus, which sits at the common carotid bifurcation into internal and external carotid arteries. Increased blood pressure in the sinus stimulates pressure reception (baroreceptors) which send action potentials to the medulla via glossopharyngeal (IX) nerve. The first CNS synapse occurs in the solitary nucleus, with relay via reticular formation to the dorsal motor nucleus of the vagus to slow heart rate and decrease blood pressure, returning it toward its normal level.

Central connections for SNS and PSNS control of the pupil should be reviewed (pages 105-108).

CLINICAL EXAMPLE 49

In many individuals, a ciliospinal reflex can be elicited. On sharply tweaking the skin of the side of the neck, the diameter of the ipsilateral pupil increases suddenly.

Discussion

The painful tweak sends a volley of impulses into the cervical spinal cord. Some of the multiple synapses there activate descending SNS pathways, which in turn induce impulses via T1 and the cervical sympathetic trunk to the eye to cause mydriasis. The ciliospinal reflex activates the same pathways as are paralyzed in Horner's syndrome.

CLINICAL EXAMPLE 50

In patients with sensitive carotid sinus, the pressure of a tight collar may cause syncope.

Discussion

Normally, increased pressure on the carotid sinus slows the heart rate. In persons with a sensitive carotid sinus, relatively slight pressure, even when exerted from outside by a tight collar, may cause stoppage of the heart beat for several seconds. This causes a blackout from lack of blood to the brain.

CLINICAL EXAMPLE 51

One of the major problems of persons suffering from tumors in the spinal canal is bladder incontinence and urinary retention.

Discussion

Depending on the level of the lesion, several anatomical facts need to be considered. If the lesion lies in the sacral cord or in the cauda equina, disrupting afferent and/or efferent limbs of the spinal reflex for micturition, all bladder control is lost, the bladder becomes atonic and flaccid, and urine removal will have to be by catheter and manual pressure on the lower abdomen. In any case, urine will dribble, and the bladder cannot be emptied completely.

If the lesion occurs at higher than lumbar levels, descending pathways in the anterolateral cord mediating voluntary control of micturition are likely to be damaged, making voluntary control impossible. The spinal reflex at the sacral level remains intact. When there is sufficient urine inside the bladder, stretch on the bladder wall initiates automatic reflex urination, almost always incomplete. In either instance, infection of the retained urine with eventual damage to the kidneys will be life-threatening.

STUDY QUESTIONS

1. Describe the different effects of SNS and PSNS on:
   a. Pupil size.
   b. Heart rate.
   c. Intestinal peristalsis.
   d. Secretion of saliva.
   e. Blood flow through skin and through muscles.
2. Define: white ramus; gray ramus; sympathetic chain; prevertebral ganglion; lateral horn.
3. What is Horner's syndrome?
4. What is ciliospinal reflex?
5. Explain how putting a drop of a solution of adrenalin (epinephrine) into one eye causes the pupil to become mydriatic, and inflammatory redness of the conjunctiva to diminish.
6. Explain the mydriasis that results when atropine, an anticholinergic drug, is instilled into the eye.

16 Hypothalamus

The hypothalamus has been called the head ganglion of the autonomic nervous system. It has a great deal to do with autonomic function, and it is in the head.

GENERAL STRUCTURE OF THE HYPOTHALAMUS

This small but important subdivision of the diencephalon lies ventral to the thalamus in the wall of the third ventricle. Its total weight is about 4 grams. It is bounded by the mammillary bodies caudally; rostrally by the anterior commissure, lamina terminalis, and optic chiasm; superiorly by the interventricular foramen of Monro; and inferiorly by the floor of the III ventricle (Figure 138).

In thickness, the hypothalamus varies from 1 to 4 mm in either wall of the third ventricle. It can usefully be divided into three parasagittal zones:

1. Periventricular region — immediately deep to the ependyma of the third ventricular wall.

2. Medial hypothalamic area — lateral to the periventricular region and containing most of the named nuclei.

3. Lateral hypothalamic area — bounded laterally by the medial forebrain bundle.

PERIVENTRICULAR REGION AND SYSTEM

A large number of very small neurons and unmyelinated nerve fibers lie near the ventricular surface to form the periventricular system. It is continuous with and homologous with the periaqueductal gray of the midbrain. An important lightly myelinated tract, the dorsal longitudinal fasciculus, originates from the periventricular system with contributions from other parts of the hypothalamus, and descends via the periaqueductal gray to send collaterals into reticular formation of the midbrain and pons, and further caudally.

This appears to be an important route by which the hypothalamus influences autonomic functions through SNS and PSNS outflows.

MEDIAL HYPOTHALAMIC AREA

In the medial hypothalamic area are found the following nuclei from front to back: suprachiasmatic, supraoptic and preoptic, paraventricular, dorsomedial and ventromedial, posterior nucleus, and nuclei of the mammillary bodies (Figure 139).

The suprachiasmatic nucleus receives direct inputs from the retina and is instrumental in maintenance of circadian rhythms, as discussed in Chapter 17.

Axons from paraventricular and supraoptic muclei extend down the infundibular stalk into the posterior lobe of the pituitary, transmitting two

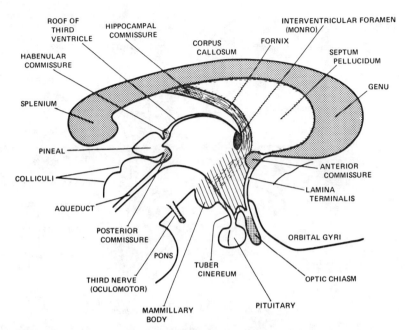

FIGURE 138. Diagonal hatching shows the extent of the hypothalamus in the wall of the third ventricle. Note bounding landmarks: inferiorly, the mammillary body and optic chiasm; superiorly, the interventricular foramen and anterior commissure.

hormones to the neurohypophysis (posterior pituitary): oxytocin and anti-diuretic hormone (ADH). Oxytocin induces uterine contraction when the uterine smooth muscle has been primed by estrogen in the absence of progesterone, i.e., at parturition. ADH controls water excretion by the kidneys.

Stimulation of the anterior hypothalamus often induces parasympathetic effects. In contrast, posterior hypothalamic stimulation causes sympathetic effects: tachycardia, increased blood pressure, and increased body temperature through shivering and peripheral vasoconstriction.

Within the hypothalamus lies a 'set-point' mechanism which controls these temperature-regulating processes. If the set-point temperature is cooler than core body temperature (i.e., the temperature of the blood flowing through the hypothalamus), the set-point neurons activate the cooling processes — sweating and cutaneous vasodilation. In contrast, if the set-point temperature is warmer than the core body temperature, as it might be if the set-point neurons were stimulated by toxins produced by bacterial infection, the set-point will activate peripheral vasoconstriction and shivering to bring the core body temperature up to the set-point. This process causes the fever of infections.

The mammillary bodies are the caudalmost hypothalamic structures. They receive most of the fibers of the fornix from the hippocampal complex and indirectly from the parahippocampal gyrus of the temporal lobe, from the cingulate gyrus, and from other limbic structures. From each mammillary body

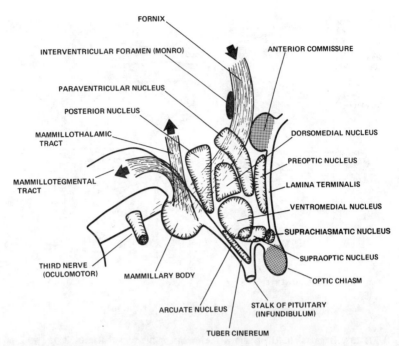

FORNIX

INTERVENTRICULAR FORAMEN (MONRO)

ANTERIOR COMMISSURE

PARAVENTRICULAR NUCLEUS

POSTERIOR NUCLEUS

MAMMILLOTHALAMIC
TRACT

DORSOMEDIAL NUCLEUS

PREOPTIC NUCLEUS

MAMMILLOTEGMENTAL
TRACT

LAMINA TERMINALIS

VENTROMEDIAL NUCLEUS

SUPRACHIASMATIC NUCLEUS

THIRD NERVE
(OCULOMOTOR)

MAMMILLARY BODY

SUPRAOPTIC NUCLEUS

OPTIC CHIASM

ARCUATE NUCLEUS

STALK OF PITUITARY
(INFUNDIBULUM)

TUBER CINEREUM

FIGURE 139. Some of the major nuclei of the hypothalamus. The periventricular system lies between these nuclei and the ependyma of the third ventricle; the lateral hypothalamic area lies lateral to these nuclei and to the fornix.

arise two large arise two large bundles of axons. The mammillothalamic tract passes dorsally to end in the anterior nuclear mass of the thalamus, relaying to the cortex of the cingulate gyrus.

The mammillotegmental tract extends caudally to the tegmentum of the midbrain, synapsing with reticular and other neurons. Mammillary nuclei thus appear to act as major limbic system relays in a complex circuitry which will be discussed later.

Control of food intake resides in the ventromedial hypothalamic nucleus, often called a satiety center. Animals and possibly humans with lesions here may eat excessively, the syndrome of hyperphagia, and become obese. The ventromedial nucleus probably also controls water intake.

LATERAL HYPOTHALAMIC AREA

In contrast to the ventromedial nucleus, the lateral hypothalamic area includes neurons whose function is to induce eating: a hunger or feeding center. Lesions here may cause severe anorexia or loss of appetite, at times leading to death from starvation.

ENDOCRINE FUNCTIONS

Many hypothalamic functions act indirectly through the pituitary's endocrine secretions. Table 18 summarizes these endocrine relations. The hypothalamic hormones or factors are produced within hypothalamic neurons. In the region of the tuber cinereum (Figures 138 and 139) these hypothalamic hormones are secreted into nests of capillaries draining into hypophyseal portal veins which descend the pituitary stalk to the anterior pituitary (adenohypophysis). There the portal veins break up into a new set of capillaries from which cells of the pituitary pick up their controlling hormones (factors), as indicated in Table 18. This system of venous channels with capillaries at both ends constitutes the hypophyseal portal system.

Two posterior pituitary hormones, the last two in Table 18, are carried from supraoptic and paraventricular nuclei in axons of the supraoptico-hypophyseal tract, and are secreted by the posterior pituitary.

AFFERENT INPUTS INTO THE HYPOTHALAMUS

Many types of input stimulate hypothalamic activity. Temperature regulation is stimulated by incoming blood temperature. Renal water excretion is controlled by the osmolarity of the blood, which causes appropriate changes in ADH secretion. Secretion of a variety of hormones depends upon hormonal inputs and feedback processes. For instance, if the blood level of thyroid hormone is high, the hypothalamus causes a decrease in secretion of thyrotropic (thyroid stimulating) hormone. Many of the sympathetic and parasympathetic activations result from inputs from the neocortex by way of the limbic system — to be discussed in Chapter 17.

EFFERENT TRACTS FROM THE HYPOTHALAMUS

Autonomic descending influences of the hypothalamus pass via two tracts that have been mentioned: mammillotegmental tract and dorsal longitudinal fasciculus. A third direct pathway is the medial forebrain bundle, a large unmyelinated tract running longitudinally through the lateral hypothalamic area (Figure 143). The medial forebrain bundle receives inputs from orbital gyri of the frontal lobe with connections in parolfactory and adjacent regions just in

TABLE 18. Hypothalamic and pituitary hormones and their interrelationships

Hypothalamic	Pituitary	Effects
TSH releasing hormone: TRH	Thyroid stimulating hormone: TSH	Stimulate thyroid gland
LH releasing hormone: LHRH	Luteinizing hormone: LH	Female: corpus luteum, ovarian steroids Male: testosterone by interstitial cells
GH releasing factor: GHRF	Growth hormone: GH	Body growth; increase blood sugar
GH inhibiting factor: GHIF	Decrease GH, decrease TSH	────
Prolactin inhibiting factor: PIF	Decrease PRL	Stop secretion of milk (lactation)
Corticotropin releasing factor: CRF	Increase adrenocorticotropic hormone: ACTH	Stimulate adrenal cortex
Antidiuretic hormone: ADH	Secreted by posterior pituitary	Resorption of water by kidney
Oxytocin	Secreted by posterior pituitary	Contraction of primed uterus

front of the lamina terminalis, with connections to and from various hypo-thalamic nuclei, and with caudal connections to and from reticular neurons of midbrain and pons. Medial forebrain bundle will be discussed further in the chapter on the limbic system.

Hypothalamic control of pituitary endocrine functions must also be recalled as a major efferent system.

NEUROTRANSMITTERS IN THE HYPOTHALAMUS

Details of synaptic interconnections within the hypothalamus have dem-onstrated that almost all known neurotransmitters occur within this small part of the CNS. These include all the 'classical' neurotransmitters (compare Table 8), the numerous peptide neurotransmitters, and putative hormones which act as neurotransmitters.

CLINICAL EXAMPLE 52

A young woman was brought to the hospital with a history of lack of appetite, loss of weight for several months, a couple of episodes of high fever without apparent cause, cessation of menstrual periods several months before, and the drinking of large amounts of water.

This is a classical syndrome of hypothalamic dysfunction.

Discussion

The four findings of this syndrome commonly accompany hypo-thalamic dysfunction: (1) disturbance of food intake, usually anorexic; (2) disturbance of water balance; (3) disturbances of primary or secondary sexual functions; (4) disturbance of temperature regulation.

Her anorexia was confirmed by her loss of weight. Drinking of large amounts of water (polydipsia) probably resulted from excessive excretion of urinary water (polyuria) secondary to ADH deficiency. This syndrome has been called diabetes insipidus, because the urine is insipid instead of sweet as in diabetes mellitus. Cessation of menses suggests a disturbance of gonadotropic hormones. In men, this effect may be less obvious, consisting of loss of erection and of libido (sexual interest). Episodes of fever without apparent cause are particularly important in making the diagnosis of hypothalamic damage, probably resulting from damage to the anterior hypothalamus.

CLINICAL EXAMPLE 53

A 38-year-old man noted, as did his family, that his hands, feet, and jaw were becoming disproportionately large over the preceding 8 months or so. He finally was induced to seek medical help when he began to develop visual disturbances.

Discussion

Acromegaly (Greek = end, large) ordinarily results from an excess of growth hormone secreted by a tumor of the anterior pituitary. If an excess of this hormone appears in childhood before normal bone growth ends with epiphyseal fusion, the patient will become a giant. When, as in this patient, the excess appears in adulthood, only hands, face, and feet enlarge.

Visual disturbances, often a developing bitemporal visual field loss, result from pressure of the enlarging pituitary tumor on the nearby optic chiasm (see Figures 4 and 89). The tumor requires immediate removal.

STUDY QUESTIONS

1. Where is the hypothalamus located?
2. Name its principal afferent and efferent connections.
3. Justify the name head ganglion of the autonomic nervous system as applied to the hypothalamus.
4. What is the hypophyseal portal system? Why is it important?
5. Name the major hypothalamic hormones and their functions.
6. What are the four commonest major findings observed in patients with hypothalamic disease?

17 Limbic System

Limbic system is a term derived from the embryonic origin of its principal constituents from the limbus (boundary zone) between the telencephalon and diencephalon (Figure 140).

In older literature, the name rhinencephalon (Greek = nose-brain) was applied, because in phylogeny the system first appeared as an elaboration of the olfactory apparatus. Its elaboration and assumption of new functions (most of the limbic system is no longer concerned with olfaction) makes this older name inappropriate.

Our ancestral first cortex has been transformed into major portions of the limbic system, the hippocampus and amygdaloid nuclear complex. Because of this, the terms archicortex (ancient cortex), archipallium (ancient mantle), or allocortex are at times applied, in contrast to the neocortex (neopallium or isocortex). Primitive vertebrates possess only archicortex. Rodents have a small amount of neocortex; in dogs and cats the neocortex somewhat overshadows the archicortex. In humans and dolphins the limbic cortex makes up only a small percentage of the entire cortex.

CONSTITUENTS OF THE LIMBIC SYSTEM

Neuronal collections which make up the limbic system include the hippocampus, amygdaloid nuclear complex, uncus (rostral part of the parahippocampal gyrus), anterior part of the cingulate gyrus, mammillary bodies, portions of the anterior hypothalamus and adjacent parolfactory area together with the subcallosal gyrus, the anterior nuclear mass of the thalamus, septum pellucidum, and habenular nuclear complex.

Review Figures 141 and 142 for locations of these structures in relation to neuroanatomical systems and landmarks already studied.

Several bundles of axons interconnect these various nuclei: fornix, mammillothalamic tract, mammillotegmental tract, cingulum, diagonal band (of Broca, who first used the label 'limbic lobe' 100 years ago), stria terminalis, stria medullaris of the thalamus, parts of the anterior commissure, and the medial forebrain bundle (Figures 141, 142, and 143).

Olfactory bulb connections have been outlined in Figures 124 and 80, from which the likelihood of functional relations between olfactory and limbic systems are expected.

Three nuclei of the brain stem project into the limbic system as well as to other parts of the CNS, and appear to have important effects on the emotional functions of the limbic system. These are the serotonin-mediated raphe nuclei of the pons (see Figures 77 and 144), the norepinephrine-mediated locus ceruleus (see Figure 145) and the mesencephalic ventral tegmental nucleus (compare Clinical Example 47) which uses dopamine.

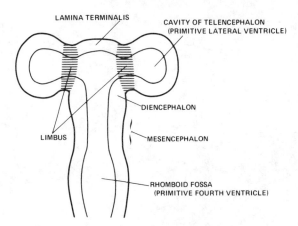

FIGURE 140. The shaded regions contain the embryonic precursors of the limbic system. The embryonic CNS at this stage is flexed. (Compare Figure 13.)

FORNIX, CINGULUM, AND MAMMILLARY BODIES

The fornix is a large bundle of fibers originating in the hippocampus in the depths of the temporal lobe, looping upward and forward around the thalamus to terminate in the mammillary body of the same side (about half the fibers) and in anterior hypothalamic and septal nuclei of the same or opposite sides. Definite function is not known, but it clearly is involved with the hippocampus and may be part of the short-term memory mechanism. See later comments on this subject. Its hypothalamic connections affect endocrine functions in certain unclear ways (Figures 122, 141, and 142).

The cingulum, another large bundle looping around the outside of the corpus callosum in the depths of the cingulate gyrus, is believed to mediate aspects of emotional reactivity. Its connections in both directions, i.e., backward and downward into the hippocampus and forward and downward into the parolfactory area and thence relaying into the medial forebrain bundle suggest that it completes a circuit betweeen neocortex — cingulate gyrus and adjacent cortex — and limbic system structures (Figures 141, 142, and 143).

Mammillary bodies relay in two directions. One relay from fornix relays through the anterior thalamic nucleus (mammillothalamic tract), thence to the cingulate gyrus via the internal capsule. The second relay from fornix or anterior hypothalamus into the reticular formation of the midbrain and pontine tegmentum (mammillotegmental tract) may be involved in autonomic aspects of emotional and vegetative functions. (See Figures 141, 142, and 143 and Chapter 16.)

MEDIAL FOREBRAIN BUNDLE (MFB)

This collection of unmyelinated nerve fibers, important in limbic and hypothalamic functions, carries both ascending and descending axons running longitudinally just lateral to the hypothalamus, see Chapter 16.

It includes fibers between hypothalamus and reticular formation in both directions, between hypothalamus and parolfactory area in both directions, from

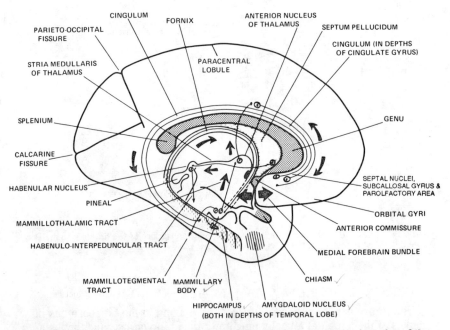

FIGURE 141. Principal structures of the limbic system as seen on a midsagittal view of the human left hemisphere. (Compare Figures 118, 121, 124, 132C, and 134.)

the septum pellucidum and, via the diagonal band, from the amygdaloid nuclear complex. A rostral continuation of the MFB connects gyri of the frontal lobe with parolfactory area, anterior and posterior hypothalamus, and thence to the midbrain tegmentum and more caudally-situated reticular formation. This connection also runs both ways (Figure 143).

The MFB is a multipurpose longitudinal pathway acting for the limbic cortex as the internal capsule does for the neocortex. In rats, it is nearly as large as the internal capsule, but in humans has been far outstripped in size and number of fibers.

INSTINCT

Instinctual behavior refers to complex functions which are built into the nervous system, that is, which operate by way of genetically determined hard-wired neuronal connections.

This is the only kind of behavior seen in birds and other small-brained animals: mating and procreative behavior, food gathering, migration, responses to aggression. In such forms, behavior can be altered only to minor degrees by learning. Our neocortex makes possible tremendously expanded learning, which we can then use to inhibit or redirect our instinctual reflex behaviors.

Instinctual behavior in humans occurs at all levels of the CNS below neocortex. Muscle stretch reflexes and withdrawal reflexes can be considered examples of instinctual behavior at the spinal cord level. Respiration and cardio-

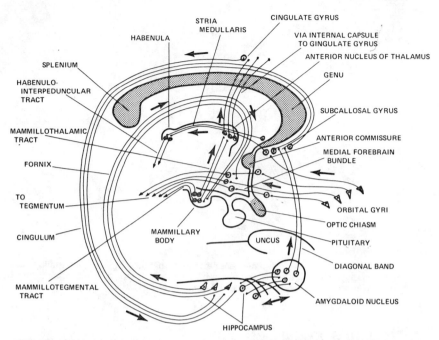

FIGURE 142. Outline of major limbic structures and connections. See Figure 124 for other components of the anterior commissure, most of which are limbic structures. Compare also with Figures 129, 139, and 141. Not indicated are multiple interconnections between adjacent neocortical neurons and the hippocampus, the amygdaloid nucleus, the cingulate gyrus, and the subcallosal gyrus.

vascular controls from the medulla operate at significantly more complex levels. The hypothalamus controls endocrine functions and the autonomic nervous system, and thereby even more complex behaviors. Each of these systems in turn influences or controls the systems lower in the CNS hierarchy.

In mammals, the limbic system is the highest level of this kind of automatic control, acting through connections into hypothalamus, into reticular formation, and into the neocortex itself (Figure 142).

REPRODUCTIVE BEHAVIOR

Sexual procreation begins with the recognition of potential mates. Primitive forms use the available distance receptors (e.g., taste in an aquatic environment) for this purpose. Olfaction, the human equivalent, is used in the same way. Sexual body odors can be quite arousing (arousing instinctual behaviors), and many humans use perfumes derived from the reproductively-oriented scents of flowers in lieu of their own.

Normal mating behavior in cats requires the basolateral part of the amygdaloid nucleus. Cats with lesions here will attempt to copulate with animals of the wrong sex, of the wrong species, or even with inanimate objects. Damage to the same regions in birds not only alters mating behavior, but disturbs nesting and nurture of young as well.

In humans, such lesions have a less specific but still serious effect on behavior, causing difficulties with social interactions similar to those seen with frontal lobotomy.

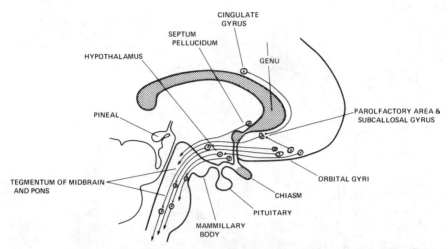

FIGURE 143. Medial forebrain bundle, simplified drawing showing only descending fibers. An approximately equal number of fibers ascend from tegmentum to hypothalamus and to septum, parolfactory area, and orbital gyri with synapses at all levels.

CLINICAL EXAMPLE 54

Phineas Gage was the classical example of frontal lobectomy. Gage was foreman of a work crew, and was tamping a charge of dynamite into a blasting hole when the charge exploded prematurely, driving the tamping rod through his frontal lobes. After recovery from this dreadful lesion, his personality changed drastically. He had been a quiet, pleasant, and responsible individual. Afterward, he lost all long-term ambition, and became irascible, foul-mouthed, and impossible to live with. These effects of frontal lobotomy (or lobectomy) are often described as the patient's inability to assess the impact of his actions. The frontal lobes appear to be necessary for an individual to become aware of possible future events. For this reason, he loses incentive (e.g., ambition), often becomes lethargic, but at the same time is irritable, and may respond with excessive violence to minor irritations.

MEMORY

Memory in normal mammals consists of two or possibly three levels. Short-term memory remains available for about ten minutes after learning. Long-term memory or permanent memory seems to have no time limit, and probably depends on some type of protein coding or synaptic changes in the neocortex.

Short-term memory appears to be a hippocampal function. Bilateral lesions of the hippocampus, either in humans or in experimental animals, produce deficiencies of memory. Electric shock applied directly to the hippocampus will often abort the experimental animal's short-term memory. Similar effects have been observed in humans after electric shock. These observations have led to the as yet unproved hypothesis that hippocampal short-term memory consists of ongoing activity in neuronal circuits (Clinical Example 42).

Short-term memory transfers into long-term memory by unknown mechanisms.

CLINICAL EXAMPLE 55

A young woman slipped on the ice and bumped her head. She never became unconscious, but appeared dazed. When she returned to mental clarity, she did not know where she was and could not recall events up to about ten minutes prior to her fall. Account for this retrograde amnesia.

Discussion

Loss of consciousness of brief duration following minor head trauma probably results from jarring of the reticular activating system (RAS) of the midbrain. The RAS lies in a narrow isthmus between the large cerebellum in the infratentorial compartment, and the cerebrum in the supratentorial compartment, and therefore becomes the physical focus of accelerating forces. In this instance the trauma was insufficient to cause more than partial loss of consciousness (daze). Loss of memory for the immediately preceding period means that hippocampal function was disrupted, so that the memory traces in the hippocampus were lost and could not be transferred to long-term memory.

CIRCADIAN RHYTHMS

Many body functions vary cyclically with a period of approximately one day. In association with the obvious 24-hour cycle of waking and sleep, homeostatic functions reflected in blood hormone levels, body temperature, blood sugar levels, and other processes vary in circadian fashion (Latin: circa = about; dia = day). Recent work suggests that the hippocampus and other parts of the limbic system may be the source of these rhythms, probably synchronized by visual inputs into the suprachiasmatic nucleus of the hypothalamus, as mentioned in the chapter on the hypothalamus.

SLEEP

Sleep, once thought of as a passive phenomenon, i.e., the absence of wakefulness, has been shown to depend upon a complex of neuronal interactions. Wakefulness or alertness results from activity of the reticular activating system of the midbrain tegmentum. As part of the sleep process, the RAS is inhibited.

Two kinds of sleep have been described: REM (rapid eye movement) sleep, and slow or non-REM sleep. Slow refers to the slowing of the waves of the electroencephalogram (EEG) during these stages of sleep. During REM sleep, the EEG consists mostly of low voltage fast activity, much as expected during the wake state. For this reason, it is often called paradoxical sleep.

Slow-wave sleep EEG frequencies vary between 3 and 7 per second, the frequencies of REM sleep between 14 and 30 per second.

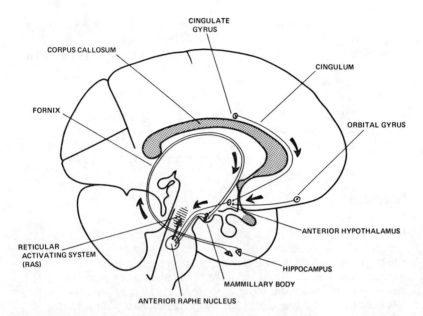

FIGURE 144. Presumed pathways through which the limbic system activates the anterior raphe nucleus for slow wave (non-REM) sleep. The anterior raphe nucleus inhibits the RAS as indicated by the interconnecting arrow.

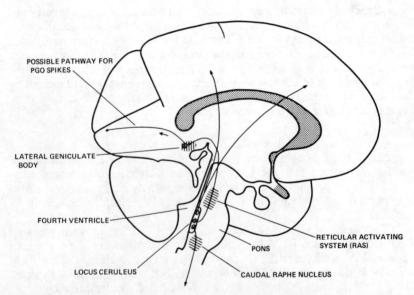

FIGURE 145. Structures mediating REM sleep. Note that fibers from the locus ceruleus travel both upward into the cerebral cortex and downward to the spinal cord.

Both kinds of sleep are controlled by hypnogenic centers in the pons. Non-REM sleep results from activity in the anterior raphe nuclei of the pontine tegmentum, probably induced by descending influences from limbic system structures. The anterior raphe nuclei in turn inhibit the RAS, and cause slowing of the EEG (see Figure 144). It is interesting to note that micro-electrode studies in slow-wave sleep often show increased rather than decreased activity in cortical neurons.

REM sleep results from limbic system activation of the caudal raphe nuclei and locus ceruleus of the pontine tegmentum. Through brain stem and spinal cord connections these centers cause intermittent rapid eye movements, muscle atony or jerking, and penile erections. They also activate the cortex and cause dreaming (Figure 145).

Pathological disturbances of sleep have been discovered to be very common. Narcolepsy, a syndrome with episodes of uncontrollable spontaneous falling asleep appears to result from dysfunctions of the control of REM sleep. Sleeping pills or alcohol induce sleep by depressing RAS or cortex directly, bypassing normal sleep mechanisms. Thus, components of sleep which seem to be necessary for its normal recuperative power are lost, and a hangover is experienced.

PLEASURE CENTERS

Electrical stimulation in humans along the pathway from amygdaloid nucleus via MFB to midbrain tegmentum or septum pellucidum may induce an indefinable feeling of pleasure. Experimental animals with electrodes in these regions may stimulate themselves repeatedly and continuously, ignoring all other stimuli, including food, other animals, etc.

In contrast, stimulation in the periaqueductal region of the posterior mid-brain, in the lateral hypothalamus or in part of the parahippocampal gyrus (entorhinal cortex) may cause a strong, diffuse, global feeling of distress, fear, and discomfort. This sensation may be related both anatomically and behaviorally with the second primitive kind of pain mentioned in Chapter 7.

EMOTION

Emotional expression is often ascribed to the limbic system (review Clinical Example 47). Various parts of the system do act as way-stations, relaying patterns of impulses to hypothalamus and brain stem to give rise to the somatic changes perceived as emotion. Emotion in the psychological sense is often thought of as purely subjective. It can, however, quite readily be treated in neuroanatomic and neurophysiologic terms, as in the following schema.

1. Somatic Responses. Emotion always includes specific kinds of somatic responses to stressful or nonstressful events. For example: pain induces avoidance, fight or flight behavior, associated with distressful or uncomfortable sensations. In contrast, pleasure is associated with comfortable subjective somatic sensations. These somatic events result from specific autonomic (SNS or PSNS) activities.

2. Perceptions of these Somatic Responses. The kinds of experience mentioned above derive directly from *perception* of events within the individual's body. *Fear:* perception of a rapid, weak heartbeat, of nonfunctioning, trembling muscles, of clammy hands *Anger:* perception of rapid, forceful heartbeat, tense hyperactive muscles, flushed face. *Pleasure:* perception of relaxed muscles, quiet breathing and heartbeat.

3. Memory of these Perceptions. The perceptual experiences become part of the individual's memory store. Often they remain associated with specific remembered events which then may become symbols of the original emotional reaction, and recall the associated somatic responses. By fixation in the memory store, the recalled perceptions of somatic responses to specific situations become intrinsic parts of higher-level function, and may no longer require the specific emotion-laden stimulus to bring them forth.

4. Somatic Responses to these Memorized Perceptions. Memorized perceptions, now intrinsic in the neocortex, may in turn induce, through descending connections via limbic system, hypothalamus, brain stem and spinal cord, the somatic changes which occurred with the original stimulus or in the original situation. One may then experience and report an emotion, meaning the somatic perceptions associated with fear, or anger, or pleasure, without any immediate external causative agent or event.

CLINICAL EXAMPLE 56

A patient came to the neurology clinic with a diagnosis of temporal lobe seizures. During his seizures, he would perform organized but illogical acts such as walking about pseudo-purposefully, taking off clothing, mumbling incoherently. He was amnesic for the episodes, which lasted up to five minutes. During some of them, he had vivid hallucinations, reliving past experiences.

Discussion

These can be thought of as limbic system spells. Abnormal neuronal activity in temporal cortex disturbs the amygdala and hippocampus, with which there are numerous connections, causing the amnesia and very likely the hallucinatory experiences. Pseudo-purposeful behavior may be the result of abnormal limbic stimulation of neocortex.

CLINICAL EXAMPLE 57

An elderly man had a CVA following which his only residual abnormality was complete insomnia. He felt absolutely no need to sleep. Where was the lesion?

Discussion

Reviewing the information on sleep centers, it seems probable that the lesion was a small one destroying the raphe nuclei of the pons. Another possibility: the rostrally-directed fiber pathways from these hypnogenic centers were destroyed by the CVA. Unless the patient has other signs of local damage, such as pupillary changes, cranial nerve palsies, etc., it would be difficult to choose between these alternatives.

STUDY QUESTIONS

1. Name the major components of the limbic system.
2. What is meant by memory? How is it mediated?
3. What is meant by emotion, functionally and anatomically?
4. Cutting the fornix bilaterally at surgery has been reported to cause changes in endocrine function. Account for this.
5. What is meant by REM sleep? Describe the physiological events that make it up.
6. Discuss the differences between sleep and coma.

18 Respiration

In medicine and biology, the importance of respiration requires perennial re-emphasis. In the course of evolution, neural control of oxygen uptake has developed the ability to respond to many changes in internal and external environments. Various chemical responses, not under direct neural control, have also developed, but will not be emphasized here.

Everyday experience indicates that humans control breathing in two ways. In rest or sleep, breathing continues completely automatically. On the other hand, one can temporarily increase or decrease either depth or rate of respiration voluntarily.

VOLUNTARY RESPIRATION

Volitional control of respiration originates in the motor cortex, and descends via the pyramidal tract, acting on anterior horn motoneurons of phrenic nerve and of thoracic and lumbar spinal cord to cause diaphragm and intercostal and abdominal muscles to contract and relax. With deep, forced respiration, other accessory muscles of respiration are brought into play.

AUTOMATIC RESPIRATION

Under resting conditions, involuntary respiratory motor activity is largely restricted to the diaphragm, often with some assistance from external intercostal muscles. Contraction of these muscles increases the volume and decreases the pressure inside the pleural cavity: inspiration is an active process. At rest, expiration occurs passively, from the weight and elasticity of chest wall, abdominal contents, and the lungs themselves.

Rhythmic action potential volleys activating the diaphragm travel down the phrenic nerves from anterior horn motoneurons at cervical levels C3, C4, and possibly C5.

These anterior horn cells receive stimulation mostly from a pair of nuclei in the medulla near the nucleus of the solitary tract, the dorsal respiratory group (Figure 146A). Axons from these neurons cross the midline and descend in the anterolateral spinal cord to the origin of the opposite phrenic nerve. A second pair of nuclei, the ventral respiratory group, lies in the reticular formation next to the nucleus ambiguus. Its axons may descend ipsilaterally or cross the midline to innervate the anterior horn cells for thoracic and abdominal muscles of respiration. They also descend in the anterolateral cord (Figure 146).

RESPIRATORY RHYTHM

Rhythmic control of respiration constitutes a prime example, and for humans a most important example of a rhythmic motor function, a phenomenon which occurs in almost all living creatures. In many cases, neuronal activity controls the rhythm, with built-in ability to respond to environmental

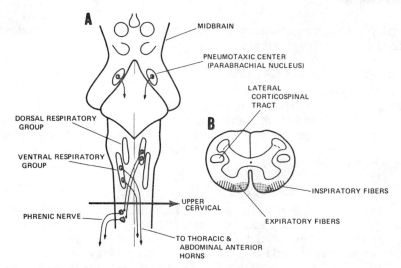

FIGURE 146. (A) Locations of medullary and pontine respiratory centers.
(B) Spinal cord cross-section at upper cervical level indicated by arrow in (A), showing descending tracts which control respiration.

stimuli. Examples of rhythmic frequencies extend from the rapid beating of cilia, to the rhythmic systoles of the heart, to the daily changes in blood levels of various constituents (circadian rhythms — see the previous chapter), to the monthly ovarian cycle of women, to the yearly cycles of birds' migration, nest-building and procreation, and of plants which bud, flower and leaf once a year. In mammals, the dorsal and ventral respiratory groups of the medulla sustain intrinsic rhythmic action potential volleys for rhythmic respiration. The rhythm of the ventral group appears to be controlled by the dorsal group's neurons. Individual neurons do not develop such rhythmic potentials. It seems likely that the basic process giving rise to the rhythms of respiration depend on neuronal interactions between nearby collections of small interneurons.

Increased levels of CO_2 in the blood, such as result from exercise, increase the rate of the rhythmic volleys arising from these nuclei, as well as the number of action potentials per volley, thus increasing both rate and depth of respiration. This is partly a direct effect on respiratory neurons. Perhaps more important is the effect on chemoreceptors in carotid and aortic bodies with afferents via the vagus nerve.

In association with increases in rate and volume of respiration, functional connections with accessory muscles of respiration must be activated. This control is probably mediated both at the medullary centers and at the level of semi-autonomous spinal cord motor neuron pools.

PNEUMOTAXIC CENTER

In the dorsolateral pontine reticular formation lies yet another pair of respiratory neuronal aggregates, the parabrachial nuclei or pneumotaxic center. Stimulation here changes the pattern of medullary respiratory activity. Pneumotaxic inputs to medullary centers intermittently inhibit inspiratory activity. Under normal conditions, this action is supported by vagal afferents from stretch receptors in bronchiolar walls which inhibit strong inspiration; an effect called the Hering-Breuer reflex.

SPINAL CORD CENTERS

As with other types of movement, spinal cord centers for respiratory activity possess considerable complexity, involving intrasegmental, intersegmental, and gamma efferent peripheral mechanisms (see Chapter 6). More or less normal respiration can be maintained either by involuntary reticulospinal inputs from the medulla or by voluntary corticospinal inputs, or by a combination of the two.

RESPIRATORY REFLEXES

Cough. Irritation in throat or trachea induces strong glottal closure followed by forceful expiration, then sudden release of the glottal closure blowing the offending material out through the mouth. Afferent inputs travel by the vagus, efferents include vagus and many other pathways.

Sneeze. Irritation in the nasal cavity causes brief palatal closure followed by forceful expiratory contraction and sudden release of the palatal closure blowing the irritant out the nose. Afferents are in the trigeminal nerve, efferents via vagus, glossopharyngeal, and descending spinal pathways probably including both descending respiratory pathways and other motor pathways, most likely in the reticulospinal group.

Sniff. Mild stimulation to the nasal cavity may induce sudden forceful inspiration.

Hiccup. Stimulation of nerve endings in diaphragm or stomach may result in reflex diaphragmatic contraction against sudden glottal closure.

Vomiting. As the vomitus is forced upward in response to organized outputs from the medullary vomiting center, respirations stop automatically. As part of the same reflex, prolonged forceful expiration often occurs, preventing inhalation of the vomitus.

Swallowing. As the bolus of food or drink descends past the epiglottis, respiration is automatically inhibited. Afferent inputs come from the pharynx via V, IX, and X nerves, and as part of the patterned swallowing reflex itself.

All the reflexes mentioned involve cranial nerve inputs, are mediated and integrated by respiratory and other centers in the medulla, and have obvious survival value.

Speech, Singing. Highly-coordinated simultaneous contraction of expiratory or inspiratory muscles, laryngeal and pharyngeal muscles, tongue and lips. Basic coordination is cortical and cerebellar.

Playing wind instruments. Similar to speech except that the larynx ordinarily acts only as an accessory wind-stop.

Cortical control of respiration such as voluntary hyperventilation, singing, or speaking bypasses the brain-stem regulatory centers. The exquisite control mechanisms which make it so easy to switch from resting respiration to forced respiration, to singing, to coughing, then back to resting respiration without the slightest problem is a wonder of automatic neuronal engineering.

CLINICAL EXAMPLE 58

A patient with a brain tumor was studied by means of pneumo-encephalography (PEG). He was in good condition before the procedure, during the lumbar puncture for gas injection, and during the first part of the x-ray photography. While being moved on the x-ray table, he suddenly stopped breathing and died. Account for this sudden death.

Discussion

With a brain tumor, there is always the possibility that the medulla may have been forced down into the foramen magnum, occluding CSF passage between cranial and spinal subarachnoid spaces. That probably occurred here, and when CSF was removed in performing the PEG, the sudden lowering of pressure from below jammed the medulla further into the foramen magnum, and cut off blood supply to respiratory centers, causing death.

CLINICAL EXAMPLE 59

A young woman was brought to the hospital because of intractable insomnia. Both she and her family had noted for several months that she would wake with a start repeatedly during the night, often with associated nightmares of smothering or drowning. Simultaneous recording of EEG, respirations, and other physiological variables revealed that when her EEG began to show sleep rhythms, her respirations slowed and eventually stopped, and she awoke with a gasp.

Discussion

This syndrome has been given the name Ondine's curse, *after the mythical figure. The patient's automatic respiratory controls were inoperative, due to dysfunction either in the medullary centers or in the descending spinal pathways. She therefore had to depend on voluntary respiration. When she slept, her voluntary motor cortex became inactive and breathing stopped. Sedation for sleep in such patients could be fatal, especially if enough sedation were given to prevent waking. To get adequate sleep this patient would have to be artificially ventilated.*

STUDY QUESTIONS

1. The expert hangman was noted for causing instant death. This was accomplished by placing the knot behind the ear so that the head was forced forward and the odontoid process of the second cervical vertebra pierced the junction between spinal cord and medulla ventrally. How would this cause instant death?
2. How is it possible for a quadriplegic patient to breath?
3. Outline in detail the receptors, neurons, pathways, and effectors involved in the sneezing reflex.
4. What prevents your breathing when you swallow?
5. What maintains the rhythmicity of automatic breathing?

Index